# Redefining Health Care Systems

## ROBERT H. BROOK

RAND
CORPORATION

For more information on this publication, visit www.rand.org/t/cp788

Library of Congress Cataloging-in-Publication Data

Brook, Robert H. (Robert Henry), 1943- , author, editor.
  Redefining health care systems / Robert H. Brook.
    p. ; cm.
  "The third section of the book comprises a series of short commentaries on specific issues, originally
published in JAMA between March 2009 and March 2012."
  Includes bibliographical references.
  ISBN 978-0-8330-9040-9 (pbk. : alk. paper)
  I. JAMA. II. Title.
  [DNLM: 1.  Delivery of Health Care—organization & administration—United States. 2.  Health
Status—United States. 3.  Health Services Research—United States.  W 84 AA1].

RA398.A3
362.10973—dc23

                                                                            2015013738

Published by the RAND Corporation, Santa Monica, Calif.

© Copyright 2015 RAND Corporation

**RAND**® is a registered trademark.

*Cover design by Eileen Delson La Russo*

### Support RAND
Make a tax-deductible charitable contribution at
www.rand.org/giving/contribute

www.rand.org

# Dedication

This book is dedicated to David K. and Carol A. Richards to honor their moral compasses, which always point true north; to acknowledge their sustained intellectual, emotional, and financial support; and to thank them for being true friends of RAND.

# Contents

# Introduction

This book provides a scientific and personal perspective on health services research over the last half-century. Its purpose is to suggest how that science base, constructed over decades of sustained effort, can stimulate innovative thinking about how to make health care systems safer, more efficient, more cost-effective, and more patient-centered even as they respond to the needs of diverse communities.

There are three models for producing health:

- The first is the classical medical model—i.e., physicians, hospitals, nursing homes, and all the other things that we associate with the health care system.
- The second is the public health model—e.g., ensuring food safety, preventing or controlling pandemics, helping communities prepare for and respond to disasters.
- The third is the social determinants of health model—i.e., understanding how education, wealth, and similar characteristics affect the health status of individuals and communities.

The science base examined in this book is relevant to all three models.

The initial essay by Robert Brook, "Exploiting the Knowledge Base of Health Services Research," co-authored with Mary Vaiana, provides a perspective on the major achievements of health services research over five decades. For example, we now know how to measure health status and the appropriateness and quality of care. We understand the link between how much people pay for care and how much they use. We know that how physicians are paid for care influences the way they practice. We know that depression is one of the leading causes of morbidity in the world. We realize that the most powerful determinants of health are not the newest drugs or surgical techniques—they are social determinants, such as education and income.

In the essay, Brook and Vaiana argue that we can make almost any reasonable health policy work if the policy takes the relevant science into account. In the current blizzard of suggestions for how to reform, refine, and redefine health care, the core facts produced by health services research should serve as a sanity check. Political perspectives may, and do, shift, but any policy that is not consistent with facts based on rigorous science cannot succeed.

The second section of the book puts a human face on the evolution of some of the core facts. In a series of stories, Robert Brook describes his personal encounters with health services research and the medical establishment. Several of the stories depict the early environment from which initiatives to define and improve quality of care emerged. This is the world before quality of care was on the national radar—before the first national report card on quality of care[1] and *Crossing the Quality Chasm*.[2]

Brook also tries to convey the context—both human and bureaucratic—in which the RAND Health Insurance Experiment team "defended" its findings in the face of strong—and often high-level—opinions to the contrary.

The message here is simple: Progress in improving health depends on more than science. It depends critically on the commitment of individuals, who must be both persistent and courageous.

The third section of the book comprises a series of short commentaries on specific issues, originally published by Brook in *JAMA: The Journal of the American Medical Association* between March 2009 and March 2012. The commentaries echo themes from the first two sections. Some explore a range of hypotheticals that might address challenges in the current health care system. For example, drawing on our routine experience with automatically updating online carts, the commentary "Do Physicians Need a 'Shopping' Cart for Health Care Services?" asks whether giving physicians cost data automatically as a part of the electronic medical record would make them better purchasers for their patients. The commentary "Facts, Facts, Facts: What Is a Physician to Do?" provides international comparisons of such factors as life expectancy, heart mortality rate, consultations per physicians per year, and the number of MRIs per 1,000,000 of the population to suggest how U.S. physicians might use such information to calibrate the performance of the U.S. health care system, increase value, and improve health.

Many of the commentaries highlight the role that physicians could, or should, play as thought leaders. For example, in "Medical Leadership in an Increasingly Complex World," Brook urges physicians to assume a role for which they are uniquely qualified: helping to define a balanced investment in addressing the social determinants of health, the requirements of public health, and increased clinical care.

A final commentary, reprinted with permission from the *Journal of General Internal Medicine*, makes explicit a conclusion we hope readers will have drawn from the rest of this book: Our future approach to developing health policies should feature big ideas and big interventions. The commentary provides examples of what such policies might encompass, hopefully pointing the way for the next generation of health service researchers.

It's time to stop working at the margin in health services research. This core message is one that clinicians, health services researchers, students, and practitioners need to hear. We need approaches that are disruptive and daring. We should use our intellectual capital and our limited resources to take a real shot at eliminating the major problems that face us, harnessing the enormous advances in medicine achieved in the last century to improve the health of individuals and communities.

## References

1. McGlynn EA, Asch SM, Adams J, Keesey J, Hicks J, DeCristofaro A, Kerr EA. The quality of health care delivered to adults in the United States. *N Engl J Med.* 2003 Jun 26;348(26)2635-45.

2. Committee on Quality of Health Care in America, Institute of Medicine. *Crossing the Quality Chasm: A New Health System for the 21st Century.* Washington, D.C.: National Academies Press; 2001.

# Exploiting the Knowledge Base of Health Services Research

The field of health services research is now 50 years old. As the United States begins to implement the Affordable Care Act, and while many groups around the world are proposing policies to bend the cost curve, it seems a propitious time to recognize some core facts that the field has established.[3, 4] This essay is intended to illustrate how a knowledge base built on decades of careful, empirical inquiry can serve as a sanity check on proposed changes both at the policy level and in the actual delivery of care.

Any viable health policy needs to be compatible both with the core facts about health and health care and with the nation's value system. We can use evidence-based truths to build a framework for changing the national conversation about health care. Ultimately, the defining questions are not whether high-deductible health plans have the intended effect, which prescription drugs should be covered in benefit plans, or why people should use health maintenance organizations. Rather, the central question is how we can change health care systems to achieve the best outcomes. How can we use high-deductible health plans where they will do the least harm, make only effective prescription drugs available, and provide care in highly organized, coordinated systems? Core facts produced by health services research should help us develop and make decisions about which policy option(s) have the greatest likelihood of achieving our national priorities, given stated constraints.

As we pursue the goals of increasing value and reducing cost growth, we need to recognize, and acknowledge, the differences between facts and values. How much the United States spends annually on health care is a fact that all of us should agree upon. How much we want to spend personally or ask our government to spend—and on what aspects of health care—involves judgments on which disagreement is likely. We should all agree about the quality of care being delivered. What level of quality is desirable is a value judgment.

## Core Facts Derived from 50 Years of Health Services Research

Here are 12 core facts that health services research has produced over the last five decades:

1. Health status can be measured.
2. Free care does not make people healthier—but they will use more care when it is free, including care that's useful and care that's not.
3. Conversely, when people have to pay more out of pocket, they proportionally reduce the amount of care they use—including both necessary and unnecessary care.
4. How physicians are paid influences how they practice.
5. Quality of care can be measured.
6. Quality of care varies dramatically by where one lives, by socioeconomic status, and, in some cases, by hospital or doctor.
7. The appropriateness of care can be determined.
8. Geography is a powerful predictor of health service use.
9. Depression is one of the leading causes of morbidity in the world.
10. Physicians and patients need smart tools to support health decisionmaking.
11. Our health care system is wasteful—but one person's waste is another person's income.
12. The most powerful determinants of health are socioeconomic.

Below we describe the health services context in which these facts emerged and the science underpinning them.

## 1. Health Status Can Be Measured

The most important scientific development in the last 50 years in the field of health services research is arguably the ability to measure health status. Fifty years ago, health status was crudely measured by whether a person was alive or dead, and age-adjusted death rates were often used to compare health in different countries. Sick days away from work or days spent in bed were occasionally used as a marker of health status. In 1965, if one had wanted to examine how the new Medicare law in the United States affected health, the most likely measure used would have been the number of days by which life was lengthened or the reduction in the age-adjusted death rate.

But a quiet revolution has occurred in what is now considered the outcome of a modern health care system. No longer is it enough to reduce age-adjusted death rates. Rather, the question has become, "Will this invention, innovation, drug, or payment approach affect how far people can run, how happy they are, or even their future health in terms of preserving organ capacity?"

Since 1965, scientists in multiple disciplines have focused substantial time and resources on developing more comprehensive measures of health. They have succeeded. Today, many aspects of health can be defined and measured.[5, 6]

Health is now known to comprise mental, physical, social, and physiological components. Measures that are reliable and valid have been developed in each of these areas. For instance, scales of mental health cover the range from severe depression to elation. Scales that measure physical functioning range from the inability to walk to the ability to run a mile. Measures of social health range from relative isolation to having multiple friends and organizational contacts. Finally, measures of physiological health assess the current function and reserve of virtually all of the organs in the body and can do so before any degradation in organ function produces overt signs, such as fatigue. For example, the amount of kidney function a person has and how much has been lost can be assessed before the loss of kidney function produces symptoms. The same assessment can be made of memory, lung function, or cardiac function.

Measures for all components of health have been tested in general populations and in specific subgroups—e.g., for people with such diseases as epilepsy or kidney failure.[7, 8]

The development of health status measures has changed the kinds of questions that can be answered reliably. For instance, in 1965, if a new drug was being developed, the question of whether the drug increased or decreased life expectancy could be addressed. However, it was difficult, if not impossible, to answer the question of whether a drug reduced the symptoms from depression, increased a patient's ability to walk or climb a flight of stairs, or slowed degradation of organ capacity. Using health status measures, we can now answer the question of whether discharge planning enables a patient to participate more fully in life in the months after leaving the hospital, or whether physical therapy or close monitoring of blood glucose makes a difference for an individual who receives these services.

Once health status measures were developed, generating innovations that would demonstrate improvement on those measures became a driving force, both for people who were trying to change the health care system and for those who wanted to produce new products (i.e., devices and drugs). For example, valid measures of physical functioning can be used to determine whether a hip replacement improves health. Hip replacements are designed to improve functioning, not to extend life—at least not directly.

Because we have valid health measures, we can assess which of two innovations is more cost-effective. We can divide the cost of an innovation into a measure of the health it produces and determine whether the innovation—be it vaccination or establishing a coronary care unit—produces more health, or less health, per dollar invested than does a comparable innovation. Without measures of health, such comparisons would not be possible.

Because we have measures of health, we can assign value to health as something more than an additional year of life. For example, we can measure the quality of a year of life for a person with mild dementia who resides in a nursing home and compare that to the quality of life of a person with the same condition who lives in the community.

The development of health measures has also raised a series of questions that society may be uncomfortable addressing. For instance, is it worth providing a treatment to someone whose health status will improve only half as much as when the treatment is given to another person? In other words, how do quality of life and health status figure into the decision of who gets what care?[9]

On the other hand, being able to measure health status has opened enormous opportunities that have not yet been exploited by modern medicine. The most significant one is that it is now possible to routinely measure the health of a population or the health of a panel of patients who are enrolled in a medical group and to use that measure of health as a way to decide what services should be provided for a population of patients and to determine whether the health objective was achieved. Reliable, valid measures of health status could be the beginning point in any medical history, physical examination, or community assessment; and changes in them could be used as way of triggering diagnostic workups, clinical interventions, or community actions.

## 2. Free Care Increases Health Service Use but Does Not Improve Health

In the health policy field, there is no clearer example of the use of health status measures than in the RAND Health Insurance Experiment (HIE).[10] Conducted in the 1960s and '70s, the HIE was designed to understand the relationship between an individual's health and how much the individual paid out of pocket for health care. Health measures were developed to illuminate this relationship.

Because the HIE enrolled people in communities that represented the American population, the health measures had to be applicable to a general population. A significant part of the HIE budget was spent developing those measures, which are now used around the world by governments, insurance companies, physicians, and the public to measure and improve care delivered in a variety of settings.

The HIE demonstrated that the amount patients pay out of pocket for care influences how much care they seek. In the experiment, people who had free care (no coinsurance, copayments, or deductibles) used about one-third more care than individuals who had some kind of copayment. In contrast, those who paid for a share of their care reduced their use of all types of services. Averaged across all levels of coinsurance, participants with cost-sharing made one to two fewer physician visits annually and had 20 percent fewer hospitalizations than those with free care. Declines were similar for other types of services as well, including dental visits, prescriptions, and mental health treatment.

The larger the copayment, the greater the reduction in use. And highly effective and less effective services were reduced in roughly equal proportions.[11]

However, more care did not equal better health. Those who had a significant copayment or substantial deductible before they received care had similar health after they had been enrolled in the experiment for five years.[12, 13]

These results were met with incredulity. Wouldn't people be healthier if they went to the doctor more often, which those in the free care plan did? Wouldn't doctors who had more contact with patients provide services that would improve the health of these patients? The answer was no.

After the HIE results were released, scientists who had worked on the study devoted considerable effort to defending the health measures used in the experiment. Fortunately, because the science on which the measures were based was so sound, it became relatively straightforward to demonstrate that the conclusions about the health effects of copayments were valid.

## 3. Patient Copayments Strongly Influence Health Care Use

We are beginning to understand a great deal more about how patient copayments affect health and health care use. The fact that patients responding to copayment requirements decrease use of effective and ineffective care at about the same rates can have health consequences. For example, when confronted with a small increase in copayment, Americans decreased the drugs they took to prevent or control heart disease, asthma, and stroke by about one-third, even though they were employed and on every reasonable parameter could afford to pay the slightly higher price for the drug.[14]

For individuals with chronic conditions, decreasing service use may decrease health. However, for the average American, increased copayments and reduced health care use might not decrease health. The reason is that the extra care used when care is free may actually produce more harm than good.[15] For instance, when care is free, antibiotic use increases for conditions that are clearly viral in nature, which are not treatable with antibiotics, and patients can develop resistance to or side effects from these medications. The use of antidepressants and anti-anxiety drugs and other mood-altering drugs increases partly for people who have diseases that could be treated by these drugs, but it also increases among individuals who have mild conditions for which these drugs are not appropriate and can cause harm. Surgery, such as carotid endarterectomy on patients who do not need it, can increase the risk of dying or having a stroke.

All drugs have side effects. The likelihood that a child will have a rash produced by a drug is related to the type of insurance the child has, which in turn relates to how many medications she or he uses. One can predict that the more generous the insurance coverage, the greater the likelihood that the child will develop a rash representing a side effect of one of the drugs the child is being given.

## 4. How Physicians Are Paid Influences How They Practice

Given how patients calibrate health care use depending on their personal costs for care, it should not be surprising that the way physicians are paid influences their behavior. Indeed, there is no way to pay physicians that doesn't influence what they do.[16]

There are three standard ways of paying physicians: fee for service, capitation, or salary. In fee for service, providers are reimbursed for each service rendered. As a result, they have financial incentives to provide more services, even if some of them are inappropriate or equivocal.[17, 18]

If you pay doctors on a capitated basis—that is, pay a specified amount for each patient they are responsible for, regardless of the level of care needed—they will tend to increase the number of patients in their practice and compensate for the increased patient workload by decreasing the amount of time they spend with each patient.[19] They also have no financial incentive to keep their practice open on evenings or weekends.

Doctors who are paid on a salary basis tend to provide fewer services, see fewer patients, and spend more time with each patient, unless someone else controls their appointment book.[20] For example, a dermatologist practicing on a salary basis is less likely to biopsy skin lesions than a dermatologist practicing on a fee-for-service basis. A doctor practicing on a capitated basis will also do fewer biopsies than a fee-for-service dermatologist.

Over the last decade, both the public and private sectors have experimented with other payment approaches. All of them include incentives of various kinds that link how much physicians are paid to how well they perform on dimensions of cost or quality—or both—that can be measured. For example, in pay-for-performance arrangements, physicians may receive a bonus if they meet certain quality targets. Value-based purchasing gives financial incentives to providers who deliver "value" in health care, where value means both the outcomes of care and the costs of delivering it. Experiments with medical homes and accountable care organizations combine new payment and new delivery approaches.

None of these payment approaches—standard or new—are inherently evil or inherently cost-reducing. But the fact that payment method influences physician behavior needs to be recognized. Publication and distribution of quality measures that assess both underuse and overuse of services that are a consequence of the way we pay physicians can be put in place to foster a health system that produces value. Just as patients faced with paying for care out of pocket find it difficult to distinguish between care that is effective or ineffective, physicians sometimes find it difficult to reduce those services that are only marginally effective or ineffective versus those things that are really necessary and important for maintaining or improving health.

## 5. Quality of Care Can Be Measured

When Medicare was passed in 1965, only preliminary work had been done in the area of measuring quality of medical care. A conceptual framework for how to measure quality had been developed. It specified three measurement dimensions: structure, process, and outcome.[21]

Structure referred to the innate characteristics of health care providers, the health system, or hospitals. For example, structural characteristics could include whether the doctor was male or female, the doctor's age, whether the hospital was an academic medical center or a for-profit hospital, or whether the physician had graduated from a foreign or U.S. medical school.

A process measure related to what independent professionals did to and for patients. Was a blood culture ordered for a person who had just presented with pneumonia? Was the potassium monitored in a person who presented in a diabetic coma? Were hands washed thoroughly prior to surgery?

Outcomes were either the general health status measures discussed above, or they might be disease-specific, such as school days lost from symptoms of asthma or seizures that occurred in a patient with epilepsy.

Initially, it was hoped that structural measures would reflect the quality of care provided by a doctor, hospital, or health system. Wouldn't it be easy if one could predict with close to 100-percent certainty that the quality of care provided by a physician who graduated from a prestigious medical school would be better than care provided by a doctor who graduated from a less prestigious school, or even a foreign school? Patients could know from whom and where to get care by looking up the structural characteristics of providers or facilities.

Unfortunately, research demonstrated that structural characteristics of medical schools or physicians predicted very little of the variation in quality of care as assessed by either care processes or patient outcomes. For example, graduates of foreign medical schools provided the same level of quality as the graduates of the top U.S. medical schools.[22] Academic medical centers may have produced better quality of care, but it was only slightly better than that of smaller, less-endowed institutions.[23] The fact that a hospital had a sterile operating room would not guarantee that a patient didn't get an infection after the operation or would not die because the operation was not performed well.

Because structural characteristics did not predict quality of care, the attention of the quality of care field turned to evaluating the use of both process measures and outcome measures to assess quality.

Just as it was hoped that structural measures could provide a definite appraisal of quality of care, it was hoped that processes, when assessed correctly, would lead to desired outcomes and could be used as the basis for quality measurement. For example, if a patient had a heart attack for which hospitalization in a coronary care unit should be recommended, the relationship between the process of being hospitalized and the outcome of getting better should be correlated and meaningful.

There is a relationship between providing medical care that is scientifically justified and health outcomes, but the relationship is not foolproof.[24, 25] Many people will get better without the treatments that science suggests should be provided. Even many patients who have a heart attack will get better if they receive no care at all. And some patients will actually be harmed if they receive the "right" treatment. Thus, there is a controversy over whether process or outcome assessments of quality are better or more valid.

However, it is true that, in general, process assessments pose a higher bar for quality of care than do outcome assessments. For example, a review of the scientific literature, integrated with expert opinion, generated a list of services and treatments that all pregnant women should receive, or at least should be offered. But virtually no pregnant woman in the United States has ever received, or been offered, everything on that list.[26] So by this measure, the quality of care for virtually all pregnant women in the United States would be poor.

However, if one judged quality of care on the basis of health outcomes, such as death for either the infant or the mother, the quality of care assessment would be much higher: Bad outcomes of pregnancy are exceedingly rare—fewer than 6 in 1,000 infants die at birth.

Most people will have reasonably good outcomes even if the process of care is deficient. But physicians believe that having good outcomes should not be left to chance. They are committed to providing the best treatment even if it will only slightly improve an outcome. To bring that perspective into sharper focus, think about purchasing a car in which the seatbelts were not correctly installed, and so they function only 95 percent of the time. It would be hard to show that people were hurt because the seatbelt only functions 95 percent of the time. By luck alone one may never need to use a seatbelt, and if one needed to use it, then it would work 95 percent of the time.

Almost no one in the United States receives what would be considered perfect care, as defined by a reasonable set of scientifically justified process criteria that could be applied to the general population. On the other hand, there is agreement that good processes should be maintained to the extent that they promote good outcomes.

So why not just use outcomes to measure quality? This approach has been pursued. The cardiac surgeons working in a number of states have produced reports that link the likelihood of living or dying after a coronary artery bypass operation to specific doctors and hospitals.[27, 28] Models have been developed to risk-adjust outcomes depending on the condition of patients on whom the surgeon operates. For instance, a surgeon who operates on a patient whose heart has already stopped has a much higher likelihood of losing that patient than if the surgeon operates on a person who entered the operating room with mild disease.

However, whether a person lives or dies in the 30 days following an operation depends not only on surgical care or hospital care but also on luck and other factors, such as the patient's discharge environment and behavior. For example, when the patient is discharged from the hospital, he might walk in front of a truck or die in an auto accident, or he might stumble and break a hip, and die from complications.

In sum: Quality of care can be measured, but there is no perfect measure of quality. Both process measures and outcome measures are problematic, and the controversy about which to use will certainly endure for the foreseeable future.

However, there is one dimension of quality of care about which there is little controversy: Quality varies.

## 6. Quality of Care Varies

The quality of care that patients receive varies substantially. However, everybody is in a very similar boat in terms of the basic level of variation. Specifically, the difference between the quality of care that the average American should receive and the level he or she in fact receives is much larger than the difference between the quality of care provided to any two Americans who differ on the basis of poverty, race, gender, or place of residence. In fact, the most comprehensive study of quality of care in the United States found that, on average, Americans receive recommended care only 55 percent of the time.[29, 30]

Many physicians and hospitals have reputations for providing good care, and there are certainly differences between and among hospitals and doctors. However, what is disquieting is that hospitals that excel at treating heart failure are not necessarily good at treating patients with heart attacks.[31] Hospitals that are good at treating children may not be good at treating adults. Doctors that manage diabetics so that the diabetic's blood glucose level is successfully controlled may not be successful in controlling the patient's hypertension or cholesterol or making sure that feet and teeth are adequately checked. In essence, the concept of a good doctor or a good hospital that does everything well is basically a myth.

Because clinicians do not produce a consistently reliable product across all measures of quality, quality must be measured in a comprehensive way in order to motivate an institution or physician to provide high-quality care. It is not sufficient to study one disease, one aspect of the disease, or one process or outcome of care. A comprehensive approach is needed so that providers trying to improve their performance don't miss important aspects of caregiving or game the system. In education, the game is called "teaching to the test." For example, if the only criteria of quality to be used are whether a woman received a Pap smear at an appropriate time, a man with hypertension had his blood pressure measured at least once per year, and pain relief was given to a patient with illness, the response of most facilities will be to improve care as measured by those markers so that they look "better." The system's response is not to improve care overall but just to improve care so that it passes the test.

As a result, if just a few measures are used to assess quality, the quality of care delivered across all patients in all diseases will be distorted, emphasizing those things that are being measured. Fortunately, we have many well-tested comprehensive quality of care measures that can help prevent this distortion.[32, 33] Such measures can be used to determine whether a policy intended to improve health is achieving its objective.

However, challenges remain to develop quality measures for other aspects of care. The most important deficiency might be measures of how well a doctor collects historical data about what is bothering the patient and the mechanisms the physician uses to turn that information into a diagnosis.

## 7. The Appropriateness of Care Can Be Determined

The RAND Health Insurance Experiment showed that more care did not result in better health. Understanding this counterintuitive finding required developing ways to measure how much a given treatment or service contributed to improved health. The challenge was to determine, based on a patient's medical history, whether or not the care rendered to that patient was appropriate, equivocal, or inappropriate.

Simply put, appropriateness is an indication of the potential benefit of a specific treatment or service. Appropriate care is care in which the potential health benefit from a medical service exceeds its health risks as assessed by the physician and the patient. In equivocal care, the health risks of care are equal to the potential health benefit. In inappropriate care, the potential risks exceed the potential benefit.

Development of appropriateness measures depended on the development of a field called evidence-based medicine in the 1980s. Methods ranging from the use of expert judgment to quasi-experimental designs to randomized, controlled trials were developed to causally relate treatment to health outcomes. Based on this kind of evidence, it could be determined whether a particular treatment was appropriate, equivocal, or inappropriate for a patient with specific characteristics.

In addition, a new field called meta-analysis emerged in which scientific principles were identified to synthesize the results of multiple studies. For example, meta-analysis makes it possible to combine results from ten clinical trials on the same subject conducted in ten different countries by ten different investigators. Meta-analysis can strengthen the confidence one might have about the effect of a treatment or procedure or program, compared with results from a single study.

One prominent method developed to operationalize the appropriateness concept is the RAND-UCLA appropriateness method.[34] It combines the best available scientific evidence with the collective judgment of experts to yield a statement regarding the appropriateness of performing a procedure at the level of specific patient symptoms, medical history, and test results. In this method, scenarios are produced that represent actual patients, and panels of experts judge the treatment the patients receive as appropriate, equivocal, or inappropriate. These judgments can, in turn, be applied to patients either prospectively or retrospectively to determine whether care that was being planned, or had been given, was appropriate. Since the RAND-UCLA appropriateness method was developed in the 1980s, it has been used in literally thousands of studies.[35]

The collective results are astonishing: A substantial part (perhaps one-third) of care given to populations around the world is equivocal or inappropriate—independent of whether care was provided in a single-payer or a fee-for-service system, whether patients had high copayments or none, or whether physicians, hospitals, or patients were subject to whatever other health policies come to mind.[36, 37, 38, 39]

As the field of evidence-based medicine evolved, it became clear that doctors do not necessarily use evidence-based medicine when they make decisions regarding the treatment or workup of an individual patient. It also became clear factors other than appropriateness influence the health care services that one receives. Perhaps the most powerful of these is geography.

## 8. Geography Is a Strong Predictor of Health Service Use

Geographic variation is an accepted phenomenon in nature. People who live near the Arctic Circle do not see the sun in the winter; those who live in Los Angeles do. The climate at the top of Mount McKinley is different from the desert climate surrounding Palm Springs. Geographic variation in climate may even help to explain why one country becomes powerful and another does not.[40]

Few expected that modern medicine would also display large geographic differences in what was provided to a patient within the same political and regulatory boundaries. But, in fact, where one lives is a very powerful determinant of the kind and amount of medical care received. For example, very early work showed that losing one's tonsils was strongly influenced by which hospital residents of Vermont lived near.[41] The variation did not reflect the prevalence of tonsil disease.

Tonsils are not an isolated example. The likelihood of receiving coronary artery bypass surgery, carotid endarterectomy, or any other fancy diagnostic or therapeutic intervention varied two- to threefold, depending on whether a patient lived in Philadelphia or San Francisco.[42, 43] The difference could not be explained by the prevalence of disease in that area.

Sometimes there is a plausible explanation for geographical differences in health care. For instance, one would expect skin biopsies to be more prevalent in areas with intense sun exposure. But why would people with the same risk factors for cardiovascular disease have rates of coronary artery bypass surgery that varied threefold depending on the large metropolitan area in the United States in which they resided?

In addition, studies consistently showed that people who lived in regions where a given procedure was performed frequently didn't necessarily receive that procedure more inappropriately. In fact, the relationship between appropriate care and volume of care was weak at best and in some cases nonexistent.[44, 45] Over- and underuse of a procedure existed simultaneously in the same geographic areas.

Here's a stunning example: Many years ago, the rate of coronary artery bypass surgery in the United States, especially in the Southern California area, was sevenfold the rate in the UK, especially in the Manchester area. The U.S. and UK systems of care were very different. Indeed, one could argue that in the United States, coronary artery bypass surgery is essentially provided by a non-system: The surgeries are performed by many different surgeons and paid for by many different kinds of insurance.

In contrast, in the Manchester region, a handful of surgeons did all the coronary artery bypass surgeries. These surgeons were salaried and practiced at one hospital, where all the bypass surgeries took place. Care was centralized, and there was one payment system. If 30 to 40 percent of coronary artery bypass surgery done in Southern

California was inappropriate or equivocal, surely the proportion that would be equivocal or inappropriate should be close to zero in areas such as Manchester, which did one-seventh as many procedures.

A study that compared inappropriate use in these two areas produced astonishing results.[46] Even though in Manchester some people were put on long waiting lists for anatomically defined heart disease that could kill them before they had surgery, the level of inappropriate care was the same as in Southern California. Geographic variation did not explain appropriateness: When the total amount of care increased, the amount of care that was inappropriate increased in almost the same proportion as the increase in appropriate care.

We live in the era of evidence-based medicine. But we cannot explain the huge differences in the use of procedures as a function of where one lives. Knowing where you live, we can make a reasonably good prediction of the types of treatments you will receive. However, your place of residence is not going to reveal whether the care you will receive is appropriate or not.

Just as disturbing as geographical variation is the fact that appropriateness, like other measures of quality of care, cannot be predicted by structural measures. For instance, board-certified physicians do not necessarily perform services within their specialty more appropriately than physicians who are not board-certified.[47] High-volume surgeons, who we might seek out because their high volume suggests that they perform a procedure better than low-volume surgeons, may get to their high-volume status by performing surgery on more appropriate people because they have a favorable referral base, or they may get their high-volume status by operating on people who do not need the procedure at all.[48, 49] You cannot reliably predict whether an elderly surgeon compared with a young surgeon, or a female cardiologist versus a male cardiologist, will perform procedures more or less appropriately.

## 9. Depression, a Leading Cause of Morbidity, Is Poorly Detected and Poorly Treated

One chronic condition, depression, which is responsible for substantial reductions in health, is often overlooked. Because of the way the current health care system is designed, mental health conditions such as depression have classically been separated from the rest of health care in terms of insurance coverage. Care for a patient with diabetes, hypertension and high cholesterol, obesity, and rheumatoid arthritis may be relatively seamless in terms of the structure of the care process. But mental health care in the United States has been classically "carved out"—separated from care of other chronic conditions.

The reasons for carving out care for mental health conditions are not immediately obvious. Some people believe mental health conditions are associated with much greater stigma than medical conditions; hence stigmatized conditions should be kept separate, in terms of both payment and treatment. Some believe mental health conditions are carved out because treatment for those conditions is very different, and relatively ineffective, compared with treatment for medical conditions. Others may believe that mental health conditions will be so expensive to treat that they need to be kept separate and managed differently from chronic medical conditions.

The validity of any of these hypotheses is questionable. However, it is not questionable that depression is one of the leading causes of morbidity in the United States and around the world.[50] People with chronic conditions get depressed.[51] People who are depressed do not perform well in their jobs, in their education, or in social interactions.[52, 53] Lack of employment and poor education decrease wealth and degrade health status.

Effective treatments for depression are well documented, and getting care improves long-term outcomes, especially for minorities, and produces major changes in wealth.[54, 55, 56] But much major depression goes undiagnosed.[57, 58, 59, 60]

If we are serious about having a health system that can improve health, we must be prepared to integrate detection and treatment of depression into care for physical conditions.[61, 62]

## 10. Physicians and Patients Need Tools to Support Decisionmaking

Both physicians and patients face considerable challenges as they make decisions about care. And the challenge is going to get substantially more difficult. Fifty years ago, the number of tests available to diagnose a problem was limited. There were limited ways to image a chest, determine a source of bleeding, or identify the cause of anemia. And the tests themselves were less complex. But given the explosion in medical tests and medicines, both physicians and patients need smart decision support tools to help them decide what should and should not be done in specific circumstances.

When the number of tests was limited, it was reasonable to expect that a physician might actually conduct and interpret some of the tests in the office laboratory, and surely the physician would know the names of all possible tests to address a given clinical issue. However, there has been an exponential explosion in the number of diagnostic tests. By 2020, there are likely to be another 10,000 diagnostic tests on the market. Our health care system already produces doctors who specialize not just in cancer or in lung cancer but in small cell lung cancer. In the future, we will perhaps produce doctors who specialize in one of 100 types of small cell lung cancer as defined by a battery of tests.

It is absurd to imagine that any human being could know and remember the names and characteristics of all existing tests and therapies (let alone the risks and benefits of each), decide which ones are effective, and determine the most cost-effective way of proceeding. Yet, assessments of knowledge and memory are still often used by medical schools, professional organizations, and state regulators to distinguish a good doctor from a less-good doctor.

Physicians no longer fill out lab slips, write the name of the test to be performed, or draw the blood for the test. Today, the doctor is likely to have a paper or electronic ordering sheet that presents all possible tests, organized according to an organ system or problem. The physician can "check" all of them in a second, even if he or she does not understand the tests, and then ponder when the results come back whether any of the tests provided information that is meaningful to him or her or to the patient.

This is a suboptimal way of practicing medicine, to say the least, but without easy-to-use help on a real-time basis, physicians have no other alternative. The same kind of shotgun approach will characterize the treatment process as doctors begin to pick their way through the use of medications. We are quickly reaching a point where the principal characteristic of the health care system will be information overload. The result will be chaos.

Medicine is just now beginning to transition from paper records to electronic medical records. Adding decision aids and guides to these systems will help doctors purchase more effective and better value-based care on behalf of their patients—and will help to solve the memory problem.[63]

### 11. One Person's Waste Is Another's Income

Waste in medicine comes in many forms, but three major ones are administrative waste, waste associated with duplicating tests because the original results are not available, and waste associated with procedures that have equivocal or no health benefits.[64]

It is quite possible that by 2025, the amount of money spent in the back office of hospitals and physicians will fall dramatically as we develop a seamless system to authorize treatments, process payment, and match patients to their doctors and health plans. It is certainly conceivable that when patients visit a doctor, they will swipe a card and the doctor would be paid immediately after the visit. Patients would also immediately pay for whatever portion of the cost was their responsibility. This type of integration would eliminate many administrative positions in the health industry.

If electronic medical records reflected all the care that was provided to a patient in any setting and if test results were available regardless of when or where they were performed, the need to duplicate tests would drop significantly. In addition, having previous test results available might change a patient's treatment. For example, if the patient's previous electrocardiograms (EKGs) were accessible when he or she visited the emergency department, and the same abnormality seen in the emergency department was present on the EKG a year earlier, then what was done to and for the patient might be very different than if the physician did not have the result of previous EKGs. Thus, the availability of information in real time might improve decisions and generate enormous savings without negatively affecting the patient's health.

Savings would result if tests and drugs that have equivocal value (when the potential health benefit does not exceed the potential health risk) could be eliminated. Another consideration is using expensive equipment or buildings more wisely—e.g., why is it that hospital and outpatient department equipment is used primarily from 9:00 a.m. to 5:00 p.m. (or, indeed, perhaps rarely used)? Using investments in operating rooms, scanners, MRI machines, and laboratory equipment more efficiently would save a great deal of money.

The enormous growth of the health system over the last 50 years has provided jobs for many Americans. It has proven difficult to outsource medical care to other countries. One might be able to outsource the reading of X-rays to another country, but it is more difficult to imagine how actual care can be outsourced.

That said, one might envision a nursing home benefit for Americans that was usable only in Mexico because the value of nursing home care in Mexico was far higher than that rendered in the United States. Perhaps elective surgery would be covered only if the operation was performed in Thailand, Singapore, or India, because even factoring in the cost of transporting patients to these countries, the value of doing the surgery in those countries was higher than doing it in the United States.

However, eliminating waste by implementing any one of the changes described above will eliminate jobs somewhere in the health care industry. There are many individuals whose business it is to bill for medical services, so making billing more efficient by automating key functions would eliminate many of those jobs. If tests were not repeated because results from previous ones were available, and if equipment were used more efficiently, then some of the individuals who make the machines, run the tests, and interpret the results would lose their jobs.

As has been the case in other industries, policies will need to be developed to help people who lose their jobs because the jobs have been eliminated. To ensure value in the health system and to prevent the health of those previously employed individuals from deteriorating, they will themselves need assistance to become productive employed citizens.

## 12. Social Factors Are Powerful Determinants of Health

In the last 50 years, we have learned that closing the health disparities gap between groups defined by income or ethnicity or neighborhood will require attention to the social determinants of health model.[65] Medical care represents only about 20 percent of what accounts for population health, yet it gets a disproportionate amount of attention. But social determinants of health, such as wealth, education, and employment, have a more powerful effect on the future health status of the population.[66, 67, 68, 69]

Eliminating health disparities entails addressing all of the issues that affect health. For instance, violence in a community leads to depression, post-traumatic stress, and low achievement in school. Providing health insurance to children in such communities might eliminate some of these symptoms and improve the children's health status, but addressing the root cause of the disparities requires curtailing the amount of violence. Indeed, it might be the case that investing in community policing and better schools will do more to improve health than providing better health insurance benefits.

The distribution of health and use of health care resources in a population is highly skewed. A small percentage of people have severe chronic disease; have suffered a cataclysmic acute event, such as massive trauma; or are born very prematurely. Over the course of a year, these individuals consume an extraordinarily large percentage of health care resources. For example, in any given year, less than 5 percent of the population may use 50 percent of all dollars spent on health care, while 50 percent of the population uses only 3 percent of the total health care dollars spent.[70]

Thus, the presence of severe chronic disease or severe acute disease contributes both to poor health status in the population and the expenditure of a great deal of money. If we want to reduce disparities in health status and control costs, we will need to find a way to treat patients more efficiently or even to prevent the occurrence of the acute or chronic conditions that move patients to the top 5 percent of the cost distribution. This might mean preventing a gunshot wound that paralyzes an individual, triggering an extraordinarily expensive lifetime of medical care costs, or controlling obesity to reduce the prevalence of diabetes, which produces a similar trajectory of high costs and reduced health status.

The fact that the health status and cost distributions are both skewed means that efforts to control costs, improve health status, and reduce disparities in health status should focus on reducing the number of individuals who have multiple chronic conditions, who suffer a cataclysmic acute event, or who are born prematurely. If these events cannot be prevented, the goal should shift to providing care in a more efficient and effective manner.

## Science and Technology Will Increase Health Care Costs

In most industries in the United States, scientific advances have been associated with both higher quality and lower cost. Computers, cars, and a host of other products are now both less expensive and better quality. However, this is not often true for scientific advances in medicine.

A few years ago, RAND conducted a study to identify the most important health-related advances that might be produced by basic science in 2020 or 2030.[71] The best scientists in key fields were assembled, and the literature in the basic sciences and clinical science areas was reviewed. Our hope was that this activity would identify disruptive changes produced by science and technology that would dramatically increase quality and dramatically lower costs.

An impressive list of potential advances was identified, ranging from a vaccine to prevent cancer to an anti-aging drug to devices to help a heart pump blood. Each of these major advances was examined to determine how it would affect use, cost, and health if it became generally available.

The analysis suggested that some of the advances would be good buys, costing less than $30,000 for each additional year of life they saved. Others were less-good buys, costing hundreds of thousands of dollars—in some cases, millions of dollars—to save one year of life. Almost every one of these important advances, which the experts saw as likely in our future, increased rather than decreased the cost of medical care.

Based on this RAND study, the reasonable expectation for the foreseeable future should be that science and technology will make the cost problem in medical care more difficult to solve—not less. Given the increased pressure on cost from new technologies, the pressure to eliminate waste will increase rather than decrease in the coming decades. Unfortunately, the scientific advances identified in the RAND work, although new and significant, were not sufficient to produce disruptive change that would both save money and improve quality of care.

In other industries, improving value has resulted from disruptive change. For example, consider the disruption in the steel industry when the method for producing steel changed radically. In the center of Bethlehem, Pennsylvania, is an abandoned steel plant, miles long and surrounded by barbed wire. It is a stark reminder of how changing technology affects both communities and individuals.

Examples of disruptive change in health care might be globalization of labor, making it possible for health care clinicians from other countries to offer care in the United States at a cost lower than care offered by U.S.-based clinicians, or providing benefits to American citizens under the Medicaid program for long-term nursing home care that were valid only in Mexico.

We need disruptive and daring approaches to fixing the U.S. health care system. Disruptive innovations are risky, but we face immense problems in health and health care. Our solutions to them need to be commensurately big.

In pursuing such changes, we need to think about their wide-ranging (and often unanticipated) effects. We can use the key findings from health services research to illustrate that process.

## How Health Services Research Can Fix the Health Care System

How can major advances in health services science contribute to improving value in health care? Here are some examples.

**Integrate health status measurement into the health care system.** We know that health can be measured. So if producing health is the goal of a health system, then health **must** be measured. Otherwise, how can we assess what we are doing on either a clinical or policy level? There is broad consensus among policymakers and providers that health has physical, mental, social, and physiological components—some positive, some negative. But currently no country—no matter what its medical care policies—encourages its population to report health status on a routine basis. Health status is not used routinely by physicians in day-to-day practice. Put another way, the fact that we can measure health is not currently an integral part of any health system anywhere in the world.

**Educate consumers to promote wise choices.** An important finding from health services research is that giving people free care is more expensive than providing care that requires a copay: People consume more care, as expected. However, free care does not make people healthier. If we are to use this scientific discovery to improve the delivery of health care in the world, then we must educate both people who will receive free care and those who must cost-share about how to better use the health care system. If almost 18 percent of U.S. gross domestic product is being spent on health care today, increasing the value we get for health care dollars spent will require dramatically increasing people's understanding—not only about health but also about how and when to use the health care system. For example, when is an emergency department visit necessary? When is a wait-and-see approach the best option? What should people do to ensure that they receive only appropriate care from their physician? How about incentives to promote healthy behavior?

Education alone might not work, and it will probably need to be coupled with incentives that are based on what we learn from the field of behavioral economics, but can we expect individuals to use health services wisely if they lack even basic knowledge about the issues covered in this essay? Can we expect clinicians and patients to have meaningful conversations about choice of therapy, quality, or value if the general population lacks such basic knowledge?

**Improve quality measurement.** Predicting whether a person will receive high-quality care is almost impossible. However, science has now made it possible to measure many dimensions of quality. Regardless of one's beliefs about how to control cost, it is essential that a comprehensive real-time system be developed and implemented to measure quality of care in order to prevent cost constraints from reducing quality and harming patients and to incentivize and reward high-value care.

Health care providers, consumers, and policymakers should apply health services tools and methods to obtain answers to the following kinds of questions so that they can use the information to improve value.

Some hospitals have enhanced the amenities they offer, at great cost, to improve patient experience. Are these more luxurious, more expensive hospitals likely to have fewer preventable deaths? Is a particular managed care organization, health maintenance organization, or accountable care organization a good buy? If a patient has diabetes or hypertension, should she receive a monthly report on her smartphone that describes the quality of care that she is receiving? All of these things are possible to do now that we can measure quality of care.

No matter how one wants to change the health system to contain costs, information about health and quality must become far more prominent than it is today. This information should be used by patients and doctors on a real-time basis to improve care; it needs to be used to correct policies that have gone wrong.

Imagine that the first thing a physician or health care provider looked at was a screen or dashboard displaying the quality of care score or the health status for every one of her patients, indicating how these had changed over the last year, month, or day. Imagine a world in which artificial intelligence was harnessed to predict potential unintended consequences of legislation, to monitor the legislation's effects as it was implemented, and to revise those aspects of the legislation responsible for the adverse outcomes and continue to monitor effects. Revisions to the policy would not require debating it again or passing a new piece of legislation. This approach would comprise a kind of continuous improvement model for health policies, creating a *learning bill* analogous to a *learning organization*.[72]

**Update information about appropriateness of care.** As a component of quality measurement, appropriateness of care must also be explicitly measured. Even "great care" given to the wrong patients (or at the wrong time) can cause more harm than good. Currently, we have no up-to-date information about the proportion of care that is less than appropriate. To estimate the proportion, we are using findings from studies done decades ago. We cannot predict who will receive or provide appropriate care. We do not know whether global budgeting or increasing patient copays increases or decreases the appropriateness of care.

Suppose we wanted to purchase individual policies in a competitive health care system that had two important characteristics. First, we could be confident that we would be treated humanely and that we would receive needed health services from a team that provided excellent care. Second, we would be willing for the policy to cover only care that was appropriate. Care that was less than appropriate would not be covered.

Fifty years ago, the science to design such a plan wasn't available. Now it is. Should somebody somewhere in the world offer such a plan? In truth, we do not know whether such a plan or such a health service exists in the world because we do not explicitly measure those three components: humanness, excellence, and appropriateness.

**Eliminate the effect of geography.** Any policy that addresses the value of health care also needs to address geography. Geography is very important in determining the amount and kind of care a person receives. The relationship between where one lives and the amount of care received needs to be eliminated by any policy that is intended to be viable over the long term. Living in Boston instead of Des Moines should not predict (everything else being equal—e.g., age, weight) how many tests for diabetes one receives.

Eliminating the effect of geography will require measuring the appropriateness of care; unfortunately, the areas that produce more care do not necessarily produce either a lower or higher portion of appropriate care. Information on quality, appropriateness, and health needs to be made available on a geographic level so that location-specific policies can be implemented.

**Integrate mental health care.** Mental health is a large component of health, so behavioral health services should not be "carved out" and separated from controlling blood pressure or treating acute infections. Perhaps policies should be evaluated by the way they integrate care and information about mental health, such as depression and substance abuse, with traditional medical care—as opposed to providing care in separate delivery systems that communicate poorly with each other. It makes no sense not to consider mental health when trying to improve physical health, and vice versa.

**Understand the social determinants of health.** The measurement of health has given us additional understanding about the causes of less than perfect health. Socio-economic forces are very powerful.[73, 74] The question is how do the systems and forces that influence health—for example, the medical system, the public health system, tax policies, and investments in public education—interact to improve health? Should policies try to remove the boundaries of such systems and integrate the approach to producing health, or should they be kept separate? Should a country develop a health policy based on fair allocation of money and on sound analyses across the many determinants of health, rather than just allocate more money to building hospitals?

At the very least, should policies try to reinforce the role of the medical system to help people achieve health when aspects of health depend on factors outside the traditional medical system? For instance, should all health professionals who see children require the child or the parent to hand them a report card at each visit, and should the message be reinforced by health professionals that the child's future health status is highly dependent upon educational achievement?[75] If it is true that people who live in places with grid cities and grid streets walk more and have less obesity than those who live in cul-de-sacs,[76, 77] then should doctors provide that kind of information to their patients so that they understand the role of the environment in affecting childhood obesity and choose residences that facilitate walking to visit friends? Should physicians help communicate to their patients that the widespread availability of food makes it difficult to maintain normal body weight and that communities should lobby to eliminate food from all stores whose purpose is to sell hardware, gas, or clothes?

Physical and behavioral health care should be integrated not just with each other, but with many other aspects of social and political life, including education and corrections. How do we merge the roles of medical care, public health, and social determinants of health into one model?

The interface of care is often the area in which quality slips dramatically. For instance, when a person is discharged from the hospital, the transition out of hospital care into follow-up care may result in a major reduction in both quality of care and health status. Certainly, the interface between people who are responsible for implementing public health, medical care, and social determinants of health is not well articulated. Policies to control costs that are directed at improving health should be judged by how directly they promote integration in these three areas.

**Foster disruptive change.** Achieving value and controlling costs will require disruption regarding how medical care is delivered and how we reward people for producing new devices and medications. For example, how can we rapidly conduct experiments to determine what level of capability is really needed to deliver dozens of services in medicine? Does one need a doctor to remove a cataract, to fix a torn knee ligament, or to advise on patients how to lose weight? If the health care system is going to be reinvented and waste eliminated, then we need to determine quickly how to address such workforce issues.

Similarly, we will need to determine whether we can motivate industry to produce new devices and drugs that extend life for more than a few months and are cost-saving. Can we change patent laws and intellectual property rights to facilitate development of an industry that would produce a different set of products?

We can make almost any reasonable health policy work if we want. But that will require paying attention to the core facts emerging from 50 years of health services research. The magnitude of the change required is so great that it is not enough to address them in a sequential manner. It will not do to spend ten years learning how to use health status measurement in clinical care, another ten years to create a transparent comprehensive system of quality measurement, and yet another ten years to develop a health system that uses its labor and financial resources efficiently.

As I argue in the final commentary in this book, what is needed is comprehensive, disruptive change—not innovation at the margins. What ideas would society and physicians put on the table if they were allowed to be creative and set aside contravening regulatory constraints? What if:

1. All communities had a health plan that promoted an environment in which all people could thrive and provided a totally integrated set of social and health services to aid people in need.
2. Competency in understanding how health is produced was required of all graduates of junior and senior high school.
3. Educational and health policies were replaced with people policies that targeted the interaction between health and education as the way to improve a community's health.
4. Many face-to-face physician visits were replaced by video encounters, encounters with computers and people in the community, or self-directed care—approaches that would be as effective as the traditional patient-clinician interaction but would lower costs.
5. Global licensure of health professionals became a reality.
6. Medical expertise was shared so that by means of broadband Internet all people had immediate access, when needed, to world experts—without boarding a plane.
7. Obituaries contained information on whether the death could have been prevented by better medical care and/or whether the death was a "good" death (i.e., whether it met expectations about growth, pain, and suffering). Researchers and patient advocates could aggregate and promulgate this information, and publishing it in this format would change the culture of medicine.

8.  Academic health centers put patients first, and master clinician/teachers became the leaders of the institutions.
9.  Expensive equipment was widely shared so that it can be used up before it became medically obsolete.
10. Men and women understood the impact of an unplanned pregnancy on their lives and, if desired, received help in ensuring that all pregnancies were planned.

We hope that the ideas in this paper will provide a kind of compass for tomorrow's researchers. More important, perhaps this discussion could motivate youth—in the United States and elsewhere—to use crowdsourcing, prizes, games, and social media to fundamentally change the relationship between people and their health care system, thereby improving population and eliminating health disparities.

## References

1. McGlynn EA, Asch SM, Adams J, Keesey J, Hicks J, DeCristofaro A, Kerr EA. The quality of health care delivered to adults in the United States. *N Engl J Med.* 2003 Jun 26;348(26)2635-45.

2. Committee on Quality of Health Care in America, Institute of Medicine. *Crossing the Quality Chasm: A New Health System for the 21st Century.* Washington, D.C.: National Academies Press; 2001.

3. Engelberg Center for Health Care Reform at Brookings. *Bending the Curve—Person-Centered Health Care Reform: A Framework for Improving Care and Slowing Health Care Cost Growth.* April 2013. http://www.brookings.edu/-/media/research/files/reports/2013/04/person%20centered%20health%20care%20reform/person_centered_health_care_reform

4. Schroeder SA, Frist W. Phasing out fee-for-payment. *N Engl J Med.* 2013;368(21):2029-32.

5. Brook RH, Ware JE, Davies A. Overview of adult health status measures fielded in RAND's Health Insurance Study. *Med Care.* July 1979;17(Supplement).

6. National Institute of Health. *Patient Reported Outcomes Measurement Information System.* Undated. http://www.nihpromis.org/

7. Vickrey BG, Hays RD, Graber J, Rausch R, Engel J Jr, Brook RH. A health-related quality of life instrument for patients evaluated for epilepsy surgery. *Med Care.* 1992;30:299-319.

8. Hays RD, Kallich JD, Mapes DL, Coons SJ, Carter WB. Development of the kidney disease quality of life (KDQOL) instrument. *Qual Life Res.* 1994 Oct;3(5):329-38.

9. Nord E. *Cost-Value Analysis in Health Care.* Cambridge (UK): Cambridge University Press; 1999.

10. Newhouse JP, Insurance Experiment Group. *Free for All? Lessons from the RAND Health Insurance Experiment.* Cambridge (MA): Harvard University Press; 1993.

11. Siu AL, Sonnenberg FA, Manning WG, et al. Inappropriate use of hospitals in a randomized trial of health insurance plans. *N Engl J Med.* 1986;315(20):1259-66.

12. Brook RH, Ware JE, Rogers WH. Does free care improve adults' health?: results from a randomized controlled trial. *N Engl J Med.* 1983;309:1426-34.

13. Chernew ME and Newhouse JP. What does the RAND Health Insurance Experiment tell us about the impact of patient cost sharing on health outcomes? *AJMC*. 2008 Jul 15. http://www.ajmc.com/publications/issue/2008/2008-07-vol14-n7/Jul08-3414p412-414/#sthash.70Xc8iYZ.dpuf

14. Solomon MD, Goldman DP, Joyce GF, Escarce JJ. Cost sharing and the initiation of drug therapy for the chronically ill. *Arch Intern Med*. 2009 Apr 27;169(8):740-8.

15. Fisher ES, Wennberg DE, Stukel TA, Gottlieb DJ, Lucas FL, Pinder EL. The implications of regional variations in Medicare spending, part 1: the content, quality, and accessibility of care. *Ann Intern Med*. 2003;138(4):273-287.

16. Berenson RA, Rich EC. US approaches to physician payment: the deconstruction of primary care. *J Gen Intern Med*. 2010 Jun;25(6):613-8.

17. Capretta JC. *The Role of Medicare Fee-for-Service in Inefficient Health Care Delivery*. American Enterprise Institute; April 2013.

18. Teitelbaum JB, Sara E. Wilensky SE. *Essentials of Health Policy and Law*. Jones & Bartlett; 2013.

19. Newhouse JP. *Pricing the Priceless: A Health Care Conundrum*. Cambridge (MA): MIT Press; 2002.

20. Sethi MK, Frist WH. *An Introduction to Health Policy: A Primer for Physicians and Medical Students*. Springer Science & Business Media; 2013 Aug 4.

21. Donabedian A. *The Definition of Quality and Approaches to Its Assessment*. Ann Arbor (MI): Health Administration Press; 1980.

22. Brook RH, Williams KN. Foreign medical graduates and their impact on the quality of medical care in the United States. *Milbank Memorial Fund Quarterly*. 1975;53:549-81.

23. Keeler EB, Rubenstein LV, Kahn KL, et al. Hospital characteristics and quality of care. *JAMA*. 1992;268:1709-14.

24. Brook RH, Appel FA. Quality of care assessment: Choosing a method for peer review. *N Engl J Med*. 1973;288:1323-9.

25. Kahn KL, Rogers WH, Rubenstein, LV, et al. Measuring quality of care with explicit process criteria before and after implementation of the DRG-based prospective payment system. *JAMA*. 1990;264:1969-73.

26. Murata PJ, McGlynn EA, Siu AL, et al. Quality measures for prenatal care: a comparison of care in six health plans. *Arch Fam Med*. 1994;3:41-9.

27. New York State Department of Health. Adult cardiac surgery in New York State 2008-2010. October 2012. http://www.health.ny.gov/statistics/diseases/cardiovascular/heart_disease/docs/2006-2008_adult_cardiac_surgery.pdf

28. State of California, Office of Statewide Health Planning and Development. *The California Report on Coronary Artery Bypass Graft Surgery, 2009-2010 Hospital and Surgeon Data*. Sacramento (CA): Office of Statewide Health Planning and Development; April 2013.

29. McGlynn EA, Asch SM, Adams J, et al. The quality of health care delivered to adults in the United States. *N Engl J Med*. 2003 Jun 26;348(26)2635-45

30. Kahn KL, Pearson ML, Harrison ER, et al. Health care for black and poor hospitalized Medicare patients. *JAMA*. 1994;271:1169-74.

31. Shapiro MF, Park RE, Keesey J, Brook RH. Mortality differences between New York City municipal and voluntary hospitals, for selected conditions. *Am J Public Health*. 1993;83:1024-6.

32. Kerr EA, Asch SM, Hamilton EG, McGlynn EA, eds. *Quality of Care for General Medical Conditions: A Review of the Literature and Quality Indicators.* MR-1280-AHRQ. Santa Monica (CA): RAND Corporation; 2000. http://www.rand.org/pubs/monograph_reports/MR1280.html

33. Wenger NS, Roth CP, Shekelle PG, the ACOVE Investigators. Introduction to the Assessing Care of Vulnerable Elders-3 quality indicator measurement set. *J Am Geriatr Soc.* 2007 Oct;55(suppl 2):S247-52.

34. Brook RH, Chassin MR, Fink A. A method for the detailed assessment of the appropriateness of medical technologies. *Int J Technol Assess Health Care.* 1986;2:53-63.

35. Gonzalez N, Quintana JM, Lacalle JR, Chic S, Maroto D. Review of the utilization of the RAND appropriateness method in the biomedical literature. *Gac Sanit.* 2009;23(3):232-7.

36. Anderson GM, Grumbach K, Luft HS, et al. Use of coronary artery bypass surgery in the United States and Canada: influence of age and income. *JAMA.* 1993;269:1661-6.

37. Bernstein SJ, McGlynn EA, Siu AL, et al., The appropriateness of hysterectomy: a comparison of care in seven health plans. *JAMA.* 1993;269:2398-402.

38. Chassin MR, Kosecoff J, Park RE, et al. Does inappropriate use explain geographic variations in the use of health care services? a study of three procedures. *JAMA.* 1987;258:2533-7.

39. McGlynn EA, Naylor CD, Anderson GM, et al. Comparison of the appropriateness of coronary angiography and coronary artery bypass graft surgery between Canada and New York State. *JAMA.* 1994;272:934-40.

40. Diamond J. *Guns, Germs, and Steel: The Fates of Human Societies.* New York (NY): W.W. Norton & Co., Inc.; 1999.

41. Wennberg J, Gittelsohn A. Small area variations in health care delivery. *Science.* 1973 Dec 14;182:1102-8.

42. Chassin MR, Brook RH, Park RE. Variations in the use of medical and surgical services by the Medicare population. *N Engl J Med.* 1986;314:285-90.

43. Newhouse JP, Garber AM. Geographic variation in Medicare services. *N Engl J Med.* 2013 Apr 18;368(16):1465-8.

44. Chassin MR, Kosecoff J, Park RE, et al. Does inappropriate use explain geographic variations in the use of health services? a study of three procedures. *JAMA.* 1987;258:2533-7.

45. Leape L, Park RE, Solomon DH, Chassin MR, Kosecoff J, Brook RH. Does inappropriate use explain small area variations in the use of health care services? *JAMA.* 1990;263:669-72.

46. Gray D, Hampton JR, Bernstein SJ, Brook RH. Clinical practice: audit of coronary angiography and bypass surgery. *Lancet.* 1990;335:1317-20.

47. Brook RH, Park RE, Chassin MR. Predicting the appropriate use of carotid endarterectomy, upper gastrointestinal endoscopy, and coronary angiography. *N Engl J Med.* 1990;323:1173-7.

48. Winslow CM, Solomon DH, Chassin MR, Kosecoff J, Merrick NJ, Brook RH. The appropriateness of performing carotid endarterectomy. *N Engl J Med.* 1988;318:721-7.

49. Brook RH, Park RE, Chassin MR. Predicting the appropriate use of carotid endarterectomy, upper gastrointestinal endoscopy, and coronary angiography. *N Engl J Med.* 1990;323:1173-7.

50. Whiteford HA, Degenhardt L, Rehm J, Baxter AJ, Ferrari AJ, Erskine HE, Charlson FJ, Norman RE, Flaxman AD, Johns N, Burstein R, Murray CJ, Vos T. Global burden of disease attributable to mental and substance use disorders: findings from the Global Burden of Disease Study 2010. *Lancet.* 2013 Nov 9;382(9904):1575-86.

51. Wells KB, Burnam MA, Rogers W, Camp P. Course of depression in patients with hypertension, insulin-dependent diabetes, or myocardial infarction: results from the Medical Outcomes Study. *Am J Psychiatry.* 1993;150:632-8.

52. Wells KB, Sherbourne CD. Functioning and utility for current health of patients with depression or chronic medical conditions in managed, primary care practices. *Arch Gen Psychiatry.* 1999;56:897-904.

53. Sturm R, Gresenz CR, Pacula, RL, Wells KB. Labor force participation by persons with mental illness. *Psychiatr Serv.* 1999;50(11):1407.

54. Wells KB, Sherbourne C, Schoenbaum M, et al. Five-year impact of quality improvement for depression: results of a group-level randomized controlled trial. *Arch Gen Psychiatry.* 2004;61(4):378-86.

55. Sherbourne CD, Edelen MO, Zhou A, Bird C, Duan N, Wells KB. How a therapy-based quality improvement intervention for depression affected life events and psychological well being over time: a 9-year longitudinal analysis. *Med Care.* 2008;46(1):78-84.

56. Wells KB, Tang L, Carlson GA, Asarnow JR. Treatment of youth depression in primary care under usual practice conditions: observational findings from youth partners in care. *J Child Adolesc Psychopharmacol.* 2012 Feb;22(1):80-90.

57. Wells KB, Hays RD, Burnam MA, Rogers W, Greenfield S, Ware JE. Detection of depressive disorder for patients receiving prepaid or fee-for-service care: results from the Medical Outcomes Study. *JAMA.* 1989;262(23):3298-302.

58. Borowsky SJ, Rubenstein LV, Meredith LS, Camp P, Jackson-Triche M, Wells KB. Who is at risk for nondetection of mental health problems in primary care? *J Gen Intern Med.* 2000 Jun;15(6):381-8.

59. Kataoka SH, Zhang L, Wells KB. Unmet need for mental health care among US children: variation by ethnicity and insurance status. *Am J Psychiatry.* 2002;159(9):1548-55.

60. Wells KB, Rogers W, Davis LM, Kahn K, Norquist N, Keeler E, Kosecoff J, Brook H. Quality of care for hospitalized depressed elderly before and after implementation of a national prospective payment system. *Am J Psychiatry.* 1993;150(12):1799-805.

61. Wells KB, Sturm R, Sherbourne CD, Meredith L. *Caring for Depression.* Cambridge (MA): Harvard University Press; 1996.

62. Jackson-Triche M, Wells KB, Minnium K. *Beating Depression: The Journey to Hope.* New York: McGraw-Hill; 2002.

63. Pozen MW, D'Agostino RB, Selker, et al. A predictive instrument to improve coronary-care-unit admission practices in acute ischemic heart disease. *N Engl J Med.* 1984;310(20):1273-8.

64. Berwick DM, Hackbarth A. Eliminating waste in U.S. health care. *JAMA.* 2012;307:1513-6.

65. Commission on Social Determinants of Health. *Closing the Gap in a Generation: Health Equity Through Action on the Social Determinants of Health.* Geneva: World Health Organization; 2008.

66. Tarlov AR. Public policy frameworks for improving population health. *Ann N Y Acad Sci.* 1999;896:281-93.

67. Smith J. The impact of socioeconomic status on health over the life-course. *J Hum Resour.* 2007 Fall;42(4):739-64.

68. Goldman D, Smith JP. The increasing value of education to health. *Soc Sci Med.* 2011 May;72(10):1728-37.

69. Bird CE, Seeman TE, Escarce JJ, Basurto-Davila R, et al. Neighbourhood socioeconomic status and biological "wear and tear" in a nationally representative sample of US adults. *J Epidemiol Community Health*. 2010 Oct;64(10):860-5.

70. Stanton MW, Rutherford MK. The high concentration of U.S. health care expenditures. *Research in Action*, Issue 19, AHRQ Pub. No. 06-0060. Rockville (MD): Agency for Healthcare Research and Quality; 2005.

71. Shekelle PG, Ortiz E, Newberry SJ, et al. Identifying potential health care innovations for the future elderly. *Health Affairs*, web exclusive. 2005 Sep 26;W-5-R67-R76.

72. Senge PM. *The Fifth Discipline: The Art and Practice of the Learning Organization*. Doubleday/Currency; 1990.

73. Smith J. The impact of socioeconomic status on health over the life-course. *J Hum Resour*. 2007 Fall;42(4):739-64.

74. Marmot MG. *Status Syndrome: How Your Social Standing Directly Affects Your Health and Life Expectancy*. Bloomsbury Publishing; 2004.

75. Goldman DP, Smith, JP. The increasing value of education to health. *Soc Sci Med*. 2011 May; 72(10):1728-37.

76. Piatkowski DP, Garrick NW, Marshall WE. Community design, street networks, and public health. *Journal of Transport & Health*. 2014 Dec;1(4):326-40.

77. Marshall WE, Garrick NW. The effect of street network design on walking and biking. *Transportation Research Record*. 2010(2198):103-15.

# Stories

I want to tell eight stories that provide a personal perspective on the field of health care quality. They describe how I first became involved in quality of care and, by way of example, track the evolution of the field from the early 1960s to the present. They also illustrate the volatile emotional environment surrounding any kind of change in the health care system—an environment that remains a powerful barrier to real system innovation.

## Story One: Why Fixing Simple Problems in Medicine Would Dramatically Increase Quality

When I was a medical student, I needed a summer job to help pay for medical school. I also wanted to spend the summer camping in national parks in the West. That meant finding a job with two important characteristics: I didn't have to do the work in Baltimore, where I went to medical school, and I could do the work competently under lantern light in the middle of the night.

John Williamson gave me an opportunity in the field of quality of care assessment. He and Paul Sanazaro had recently completed a study in which they asked a random sample of physicians at academic medical centers to describe an incident that embodied either good or bad care. These descriptions, which had been transcribed on standard-size paper, represented over 10,000 descriptions of what these talented physicians deemed good and bad care. John tried to persuade medical students to code these descriptions for analysis, but most students evidenced no interest.

I thought these descriptions represented a great opportunity. I could put the 10,000 pieces of paper in the trunk of my car, check out every medical text I thought I would need to code the descriptions, and embark on a tour of the national parks in the western United States. John's only requirement was that all the examples had to be coded by the time school began in September.

I disappeared for the summer and spent my time at night coding the descriptions. To my amazement, I did not need to refer to a single one of the medical textbooks I had brought with me. Even though I had virtually no clinical experience, I quickly discovered that I didn't need much clinical background to understand what the leading professors in academic medical centers thought was good or bad care.

The descriptions went something like this:

- "I decided to go down to the X-ray department and look at the X-ray with the radiologist, and, to my amazement, I discovered that there was a significant lesion on the X-ray that wasn't included in the report."
- "I was actually awake in the middle of the night and saw a low potassium reading on a patient. I prevented the patient from dying by giving him potassium."
- "I saw a patient who had not been called regarding an abnormal X-ray. By the time the patient came back to see the physician, the tumor was no longer resectable."

These brilliant physicians were describing the simplest types of medical errors. If some of the errors were rectified in follow-up or by looking at a test in a timely manner, then they were considered an example of good quality of care. If the errors were not remedied, then they were considered an example of poor quality of care. The problem for me as a young medical student was that not a single lecture or class I had been exposed to had anything to do with what I had just spent my summer learning. Quality of care in medical school was all about the brilliant diagnostician, the insightful diagnosis, the innovative use of some drug, or something at the far borders of surgical innovation. That is the kind of quality of care celebrated in the clinical years. No one taught us that if we just fixed the simple problems in medicine, quality of care might actually increase dramatically and the health outcomes of our patients might be significantly better.

Fast-forward almost 50 years. We are still talking about how to fix simple problems: how to get physicians to wash their hands; how to make sure we use a standardized protocol and insert a central venous line so that it does not become infected; how to handle a catheter that goes into the bladder so that it does not produce an infection; how to make sure that we see abnormal laboratory tests and act on them in a timely manner.

After half a century, medicine has still not figured out how to solve simple problems that were identified over 50 years ago by leading educators in the United States.

## Story Two: Whom Does the Institutional Review Board Protect?

Internship and residency anywhere in the United States, and of course at Johns Hopkins, was very demanding. The patients we had were our patients, and we were expected to provide 24/7 care for them. I remember having a conversation with one of my fellow interns, who was feeling guilty that he was going to take six hours off on his wedding day. He had a patient who was unstable, and he wanted me to cover for him.

The purpose of this story is not to suggest that the workload expectations for interns and residents were inappropriate or that they were not conducive to learning more about patient care. Rather, I want to raise a different and even more difficult issue—that is, did anything we do make a difference?

After one very difficult month in the emergency department in which we all had worked extremely hard, I was awakened one evening by a voice that asked, "Did I really do any good in my last emergency shift?" In those days, when people came to the emergency department with a complex problem that didn't require immediate hospitalization, we would do a two- or three-hour workup and conduct extensive tests to determine what we should do for the patient.

Of course, if these tests were to have any value, they required follow-up. I had the idea that it would be useful to contact patients six months after their emergency department workup and ask them simple questions about what had happened to them in order to understand what we did right and what we did wrong. My hope was that I could demonstrate that the hard work we did was extremely worthwhile and that patients' lives and their health trajectories had been changed for the better by the work we had done.

To my amazement, I found the opposite. When I tracked down these patients, in the process acquiring tracking skills that I think would have done the CIA or FBI proud, I found that many of the patients had been lost to follow-up. Many had never returned for a follow-up visit. Even more important, we had made it almost impossible for patients to get follow-up after they left the emergency department. They had to schedule their own visit, which often meant being on hold on the telephone for an interminable amount of time. If they missed their appointment for any reason—the weather in Baltimore was bad and the streets were not passable, or they could not leave a sick child at home alone, etc.—they had to go back to the emergency department and begin the whole process again—maybe even receiving a new, mostly unnecessary, workup for the same problem. There was no way they could simply talk to somebody and get back into the system.

Based on this simple study, I suggested to the CEO of Johns Hopkins that they might want to hire someone for the emergency department who could help arrange appointments before the patient left the emergency department or provide at least a minimum amount of care coordination. Almost a quarter of a century later, I received a note from a new CEO that basically said, "Oh, by the way, we finally adopted your idea and hired the kind of person you described to help coordinate care."

It took a quarter of a century to implement a very simple change that would help physicians follow up with patients and provide quality care to them.

Of course, nobody knows whether that change was implemented efficiently and effectively, and the study I did 50 years ago has not been repeated. But if it were, I wouldn't be surprised if most patients seen in the emergency department were still lost to follow-up in a relatively short period of time; thus, quality of care provided in the emergency department becomes irrelevant over time because of lack of follow-up—i.e., the good done in the emergency department is attenuated by a lack of follow-up care.

For me, the results of the patient follow-up effort 50 years ago have raised a number of ethical questions. For example: If your emergency department delivers fine clinical care, but you do not provide follow-up after the patient leaves the emergency department, is the emergency department really good? In addition, if you have a really good emergency department and admit patients to a hospital that is not good, can you call the care in the emergency department good even if the hospitalized patient will have a poor outcome?

In the 1960s, I decided to publish the study results, identifying the hospital in which the study was done. After the editor of the *New England Journal of Medicine* accepted the publication, which required my enduring his many assertions that I could not write in the English language, he wrote a letter to the dean of the Johns Hopkins University School of Medicine informing the dean that he would publish the study only if the dean signed a letter holding the journal harmless from any liability resulting from publishing the study.

At that time, David Rogers was dean of the medical school. He looked at the letter, signed it, and sent it back. The article was published. I wonder if today's deans would do the same.

Wanting to counter this image, the hospital administrator invited reporters to see the emergency department. It was brand new and was the best emergency department in the city at the time. However, no one had told the physicians who were on duty that reporters were coming by. As the hospital administrator and the reporters swung open the double doors to the emergency department, the first thing they saw was a woman running around totally nude, followed by a physician who had not shaved for four days because he was on duty during the holidays. He had a stethoscope at the ready because he was trying to make sure there was nothing wrong with the patient physically before he was willing to sign papers to commit the patient to a mental institution. Needless to say, the hospital administration did not have warm, fuzzy feelings about me.

There are multiple lessons to be learned from this experience. First, following up with patients is critical. Every intern, resident, and physician needs to know what happens to their patients if they are going to improve their performance or learn what therapies work or don't work. But, to this day, providing such information does not occur. In fact, knowing what happens to their patients may be the number one priority for today's interns and residents.

Second, transparency is important, but given the kind of experiences described above, it's an uphill battle to increase it quickly. Physicians still don't have a comfortable relationship with the press or the transparent reporting of results from their institutions. It would have made such a difference if the follow-up study had been published in a world where transparency was an already established fact—a world where all deaths were assessed as to whether they were preventable or not, and, after patient privacy was protected, the public would know for each institution the proportion of deaths that were preventable or not preventable, and the reporting of such data would be done in a compassionate and caring but still informative way. That kind of transparency has yet to be achieved, except in a few cases.

In retrospect, the biggest hurdle in doing these kinds of follow-up studies turned out to be getting institutional review board (IRB) approval. As a naïve resident, I thought the purpose of an IRB was to protect the patient. What I discovered was that the role of the IRB was to protect the reputation of institutions as well, and a physician/researcher following up with patients to see what had happened to them was considered scary and dangerous to the institution's reputation, even though it might benefit the patients by reconnecting them to care.

## Story Three: Introducing Quality Measurement to the Wild West

When I completed my residency, I was lucky enough to take a job in the Public Health Service, in the organization that would eventually become the Agency for Healthcare Research and Quality but was then called the National Center for Health Services Research. The center had an ambitious, forward-looking agenda. One part of that agenda was to establish area-wide medical care review organizations that would report quality of care on an area-wide basis. When the center began this work, I thought that states like Massachusetts, Connecticut, and New York might become the first experimental medical care review organizations, and that the academic medical centers in these states, which were the best in the world, would become the first institutions to actively support such an activity. I was amazed when Mississippi, Georgia, and Albemarle County in Virginia were designated as places where the program would begin.

The physicians who undertook leadership roles were amazing, unassuming but dedicated individuals. Here are several examples of what they had to contend with.

In Albemarle County (the home of Thomas Jefferson), I went to a meeting at which the leaders of the local experimental medical review organization were explaining what they were about to the Albemarle medical society. Before the speaker could say more than five words, a physician in the back of the room got up, singing "The Star-Spangled Banner." He put his hand over his heart, pledged allegiance to the flag of the United States, and called the speaker a communist, and all the physicians walked out of the meeting. I was stunned. However, to my amazement, the leader of this program said, "That's what I deal with, and I will eventually succeed."

My next experience was in Mississippi. This was the early 1970s, and I went down to the Delta region to talk to the physician who was attempting to establish an experimental medical review organization in the state. He was a family practitioner whose first name was Mildred. I walked into his office and sat down. I was trying to understand why this particular physician would begin an experimental medical care review organization. When I asked that question, he said, "Bob, there were two physicians in my office yesterday who asked the same question—but they were not sitting down. They were standing where you are now sitting, and they were wearing gun belts with two six-shooters in each belt, and they said to me, 'Mildred, what do you think you're doing?'" I was waiting for Mildred to answer that question, but after a long pause, I asked, "What happened next?" Mildred turned to me calmly and said, "I asked them to read the certificate that hangs over the patient bed in my examining room." In his office, there was a desk and an examining facility in one large room. When I entered the office, I had not seen the certificate over the patient bed, so I got up to read it. As I was walking over to the bed, I could not imagine what could be on that certificate that would have convinced those two physicians to go home, keep their guns in their holsters, and not provoke any more trouble. I was amazed to discover that the only certificate he had in his examining room stated that he was a three-time past president of the Mississippi Gun and Rifle Association. Apparently, that was enough for the physicians; they left.

The beginning of the quality of care field was tempered by these kinds of concerns.

New Mexico also had an experimental medical care review organization. Part of what that organization did was examine claims from the Medicaid program to understand which doctors were prescribing what medications. They discovered that a few doctors were prescribing a large percentage of narcotic medications in the state, and it didn't seem like they had patients who needed palliative care. The physician leaders knew they had to do something, but they were actually frightened about how to do it.

After a conversation with the leaders of the medical care review organization, I thought that the best strategy might be to find a public place to show the physicians that we knew about their activities. Since these physicians lived in rural New Mexico, we calculated that the best time for a meeting would be around five in the morning at a local diner where all the farmers or ranchers came before they went out to do their work. We thought that if the place was packed, there would be little opportunity for violence, and our lives would not be in jeopardy.

So one day we walked into the diner to meet with the doctors over breakfast. We carried in huge books of IBM printouts to show the physicians what their prescribing profiles looked like. The tactic worked. None of us were injured. There was no screaming, no violence. At the end of the day, the physicians knew that they would have to change their behavior.

## Story Four: Passionate Responses to the Notion of Change

When I came to UCLA/RAND to work on the RAND Health Insurance Experiment (HIE), part of my job was to convince medical societies not to obstruct the experiment and to permit it to operate on their site. One of the study sites was in Dayton, Ohio, and we arranged a lunch meeting with the leaders of the medical society there. Things seemed to be going pretty well until one of the physicians rose and read an excerpt from Edward Kennedy's proposal for universal health insurance in the United States. He then alleged that we were a stalking horse for Kennedy, accused us of being communists, and commanded us to leave. We left. Needless to say, we were somewhat shaken by this hostile reception.

But, to our amazement, even after this episode, virtually all the physicians in Dayton were willing to be part of the experiment—i.e., physicians received money from the insurance company we had established for the experiment with government funds and for providing care to the patients enrolled in the experiment.

After Dayton, we flew to Seattle, Washington, where we were trying to enroll Group Health Cooperative in the experiment as a managed care provider to whom we could randomly assign families living in Seattle who had previously received fee-for-service care. We had arranged a dinner meeting to discuss their participation in the experiment. As in Dayton, the meeting appeared to be going well. However, as we were about to leave, several physicians rose and denounced us as fascists. They accused us of conspiring with the U.S. government, which did not want to provide universal health care. Instead, they said that the U.S. government was going to fund an experiment that would permanently delay the likelihood that everyone would get health insurance by a decade or more.

In the space of less than 12 hours, we had been called both communists and fascists, by two different groups of physicians. Luckily, we were able to get out of town. I assure you that on the way back to Los Angeles, alcohol was very appealing.

What I learned from this experience is that getting people to cooperate and participate in work that requires change in health system design may be much harder than getting physicians and organizations to collaborate in testing one drug versus another or one medical device versus another. The notion of changing the health care system elicits enormously strong feelings, both pro and con. Those feelings have not changed in their nature or intensity.

The HIE could have been followed with a series of randomized trials that would have assessed how variations in care delivery affect quality and health. Unfortunately, the HIE stands out as a well-known and widely cited anomaly in the history of science rather than as an activity that led to additional experimental studies that in turn led to the production of sound empirical evidence about the health effects of major innovations in health system design.

Stories such as these illustrate the kinds of passionate responses that health system innovation of any kind provokes. In moving forward with implementation of health care reform, we would be wise to understand the nature of the forces at play.

## Story Five: Why Free Care Doesn't Improve Health

The Health Insurance Experiment allowed us to draw conclusions about how the size of an individual's coinsurance or deductible affected health. As the leading physician on the study, I spent a great deal of my time in the next few years trying to communicate these results to a variety of audiences.

Simply put, the HIE used a randomized clinical trial design in six communities in the United States to determine how providing people free care instead of care that they had to pay something for when they received it affected their health status. When I had helped to design the experiment many years earlier, I expected that providing people free care would encourage them to seek out their physician when they needed care and that the care provided would increase the likelihood that individuals would get healthier faster. In other words, free care would produce more health care, but that in turn would improve health and result in fewer hospitalizations.

To my amazement, this did not occur. Allowing people to go to physicians without having to pay anything up front did significantly increase the amount of care they used. However, at the end of the experiment, the health status of people who had been enrolled in the free care plan was no better than the health of people enrolled in one of the cost-sharing plans. It was left to me to try to defend that result.

Fortunately, we had spent an enormous amount of money in the experiment measuring every dimension of health status that could conceivably be measured, and, therefore, our results were pretty airtight. Nonetheless, I was amazed at people's unwillingness to believe the results. Of course, they believed the result that people would use more care when care was free, but they also believed that more care would improve health. In fact, we had demonstrated that getting more care may involve getting care that was not needed and thus actually do more harm than good.

Fast forward many years. We are still debating the value of care, such as screening for prostate disease or even breast cancer. We question whether such screenings identify people who will never get serious forms of those diseases but who suffer a great deal as a result of screening because they undergo unnecessary procedures and operations.

## Story Six: Age and Resistance to Change

After the HIE demonstrated that free care did not improve health, we explored the hypothesis that this result reflected two types of care that an individual received from a physician: One type of care was clearly appropriate in that the health benefit of receiving the care was greater than the health risk of receiving it. The other type of care was either equivocal or inappropriate—that is, the health benefit and the health risk were about the same, or the health risk exceeded the health benefit.

We developed a way to measure appropriateness of care and applied it to assess care in places throughout the world. We found that perhaps one-third of the care provided was either clearly inappropriate or, at the very best, produced no net benefit over the risk that it posed.

These assessments were done in an era when medicine was beginning to change rapidly. In addition, the control of medicine was shifting from individual hospitals and individual physicians to large for-profit firms that were taking over the practice of medicine. We wondered aloud whether we could change the direction and control of this evolution and increase the likelihood that physicians would still control medicine. We thought that if the American Medical Association (AMA) came out with a statement that physicians should be responsible for the appropriateness of the care they provided and that physicians should be accountable for providing only appropriate care, then the organizational structure and management of health care might not shift toward the large for-profits.

Believing this to be the case, we presented the results of our appropriateness work to the board of governors of the AMA, and, to our amazement, virtually all of the members of the board agreed. It looked like they would take this proposition to the House of Delegates. However, one physician—the oldest physician on the board—stood up and said, "Nothing really will happen in five years, and, by that time, I will not be practicing medicine anymore. Therefore, I would like to table this motion indefinitely." And that's what the board decided to do, since the general operating principle was that taking something to the House of Delegates required agreement of the entire board.

This statement about age should be not taken to suggest that the older a physician is, the less willing he or she is to agree to change the practice of medicine. In one of the previous stories, I described the experimental medical care review organizations as a forerunner of organizations that were established to improve quality of care. Their implementation was largely determined by another past president of the AMA, who was also the oldest person in the room. His remark to his much younger colleagues when they were considering whether to change the way quality of care was being assessed went something like this: "I am by far the oldest person in the room, and I'm willing to try something new. Why are you so scared of change?" The change being debated was to assess quality of care on an area-wide basis, on a geographic basis, or in a state or a city, instead of just within a given institution. This shift in focus has made all the difference in the world in trying to move the quality improvement movement forward.

## Story Seven: Resisting Funder Pushback When Findings Don't Match Expectations

One of the studies I was lucky to be part of examined, at a clinical level, the impact of changing the way we pay for hospital care from cost-plus to a fixed price. Today, that's known as paying for care by diagnostic related groups (DRGs). People believed that if you changed the way you paid for care, there would be big changes in patients' length of stay in the hospital, and perhaps quality of care as well. Up to the time we did our study, there was no national clinical study of how changing payment methods affected quality and outcomes of care. We organized a sophisticated, national before-and-after study to assess the impact of this policy change. The study was paid for by the U.S. government using taxpayer dollars.

We found that, almost overnight, hospitals and physicians reacted to the change in payment policy by decreasing hospital length of stay by almost one day; we also found that, in general, quality of care in the hospital was the same or even slightly improved. However, people were discharged from the hospital sicker and quicker, potentially impacting their subsequent health. We also found that many of the patients discharged from the hospital did not have even rudimentary discharge plans. We told the government that we would publish these results.

They were concerned—perhaps overly so—that publishing the results might produce an uproar about the implementation of the DRG fixed-cost payment program that they had implemented nationwide under Medicare. We were literally warned by our government that if we published the results we would never receive government funding again. Of course, we published the results, and relationships with the government were cool. Even our wimpy suggestion that the analysis should be repeated to determine if the same outcomes were reproduced was never funded.

There is currently a lot of concern by journal editors regarding funding sources and how they may bias the presentation of results. Having received money from almost every funding source, I agree with that concern. However, the accepted wisdom is not true. For-profit funders, such as pharmaceutical companies, are not the only ones that pressure researchers when results come out in ways that funders don't like. Whether money comes from foundations, the government, or for-profit firms, any time you report a result that goes contrary to the funder's belief, you can expect a reasonable amount of pressure to retract or not publish the results. There are many stories that could be told to illustrate this sad truth. But the one I find hardest to accept is the one in which our government is responsible for such behavior.

Of course, none of these behaviors are universal, and there are many examples of courageous funders who are willing to see in print that their products or ideas did not produce positive change.

## Story Eight: Transparency and Responsibility

The final story describes both an extraordinarily courageous high-ranking government official and another such official who was not. The first profile involves the issue of transparency of patient outcome results. Today there is an enormous amount of information about how well hospitals—and, in some cases, physicians—perform. Performance is measured using a variety of metrics. But that was not always the case.

Many years ago, a method was developed to predict differences, after controlling for the patient's condition, in the ability of the hospital to keep a person alive who was being treated for a variety of conditions. It was possible to demonstrate that hospitals treating patients with heart attacks, pneumonia, stroke, or many other conditions had different death rates, even after adjusting for the types of patients they treated—e.g., how sick the patient was or how many other conditions the patient had. The question was what to do with such data and whether to trust the American people to interpret them appropriately.

I participated in a meeting in which there were only four people in the room. One was a high-ranking government official. The second was the president of the American Hospital Association (AHA). The third was the president of the AMA. The goal of the government official was to gently communicate to the presidents of the AHA and the AMA that he was going forward with a policy that reported, by hospital name, these differences in death rates. My job, as it turned out, was to be the methods expert.

Every time an objection was made by the head of the AMA or the AHA, the government official would turn to me and say, "Bob what do you think about that?" and I would try to produce the best scientific answer I could. More times than not, the science suggested that it was better to go forward with reporting such results than not reporting them.

The meeting was over in about an hour, and I literally became *persona non grata* to the AMA and the AHA almost overnight, but I am happy to say that the movement toward increased transparency began the next year. The government's publication of these comprehensive results has led to enormous activity over the ensuing years to increase the transparency of health care.

On the other hand, at about the same time, I also participated in a meeting that did not go so well. Early on in the AIDS epidemic, RAND had done some clinically detailed work that examined the spread of HIV among people. We used that work to estimate the impact that HIV and AIDS would have in the United States and came up with numbers of deaths that were much, much higher than the conventional wisdom. At the same time, there was growing awareness that there might be public health measures that could help slow the HIV epidemic.

We had the opportunity to present our results to a group of very high-ranking health officials in Washington, D.C. It was the last meeting of the day, and people were tired. We walked into the room, and as we were sitting down we were asked a question about the number of cases of AIDS that we thought would occur in the United States. The current wisdom was that the epidemic would peak, disappear, and affect very few people. We cited a very large number that actually turned out to be an underestimate of what happened in the United States. Before we could even sit down, the chairman of the meeting said, "Thank you very much, the meeting is over, it never occurred, and we are all dismissed." It was a long time before the government was motivated to do something that would be effective in controlling the AIDS epidemic.

## Conclusion

The goal of sharing these stories is not to blame people or to retroactively question people's judgment and wisdom. Rather, it is to illustrate to those who are trying to produce new knowledge about the U.S. health care system that it is not all about left-brain research designs and choosing the proper statistical technique. The impact of one's work will have a lot to do with how it's sold and distributed to people. If we are going to increase the likelihood that the work will be used to make appropriate changes in people's health, we will need to catch up with all of the advances in social media and communication that have occurred in the last five years. It is also important to use such media to tell these kinds of stories not 30 years after they occurred but as they are occurring. We need to figure out how to combine storytelling with hard science in a way that produces change for the good. That will be the challenge of the future.

# Commentaries

The following commentaries, published between March 2009 and March 2012, echo some of the themes highlighted in the first two sections of this book. For example, some of them explore hypothetical policies that might address challenges in the current health care system. Others highlight what role physicians could play as thought leaders and argue why future health services research needs big ideas and big interventions.

The commentaries are reproduced here with the kind permission of *JAMA: The Journal of the American Medical Association* and the *Journal of General Internal Medicine*.

# Quality, Transparency, and the US Government

*Robert H. Brook, MD, ScD*
JAMA, *April 1, 2009—Vol. 301, No. 13, pp. 1377–1378*

Some solutions for producing a better health care system in the United States and abroad call for paying clinicians more for better performance. For this solution to work, valid and reliable measures of performance must be available. Although the quality-of-care field has matured and many such measures have been produced, a need for better methods and indicators by which performance can be assessed remains.

In 2001, the government of California, responding to calls to improve quality of care, decided to produce routinely available statewide reports on mortality following isolated coronary artery bypass surgery, by hospital and physician.[1] The outcome-reporting program is housed in the Office of Statewide Health Planning and Development. I was asked to chair the committee that oversees the production of these reports, the purpose of which is to increase public and professional knowledge about this procedure.

Committee members include health services researchers, cardiologists, and cardiac surgeons, all of whom serve without compensation except for travel reimbursement. All activities of the committee are documented in the public domain.[2] All committee meetings are announced, as is the agenda,[3] and anyone wishing to attend a meeting is welcome to do so. Every decision and every vote of the committee is taken in public. Issues such as "What is an isolated coronary artery bypass surgery?" which may involve technical details such as "How many staples in the lung disqualify the operation from being isolated?" or "When is a mesh a mesh?" or "What really is the first laboratory reading on creatinine in a patient's medical record?" are all discussed and debated. So are the statistical methods to be used in adjusting the outcome for differences in-patient and disease characteristics, the outcomes to be selected, the method for auditing the data, and even the format for displaying the data in the final report. Nothing is discussed or decided in secret.

The committee has voiced frustrations including wanting to see the process made more efficient and more effective and wanting more timely produced results. Ongoing efforts to persuade the state to provide additional resources to improve the reports and to broaden the committee's scope to other cardiac procedures or to other dimensions of quality such as the appropriateness of the use of coronary artery bypass surgery were mostly unsuccessful.

However, over time, the wisdom of the committee has become evident, and the patience of its members, myself excluded, is legendary. Any surgeon has the right to appeal the results of the report and appear before the committee. The grace, elegance, and preparation of the cardiologists and cardiothoracic surgeons on the committee are extraordinary. So even though the committee would like the report to be broader and better, it is the outcome of a public process with all of the benefits of transparency in a democratic society.

This experience with the outcome-reporting committee contrasts sharply with some policies pursued by the federal government. The federal government last year decided to develop better measures of quality of care and issued a request for proposals to which qualified institutions could respond.[4] In the statement of work for the contract, the Centers for Medicare & Medicaid Services (CMS) identified specific quality improvement strategies, including collaboration with private- and public-sector partners, publication of quality measurements and information for both beneficiaries and health professionals, a payment system that rewarded quality, promotion of health information technology, and active partnerships to bring effective innovations to patients rapidly and to monitor the effectiveness of technologies for which CMS was already paying.

In a time of substantial budget stress, investing in measures of quality of care is brave. The decision signals that at least the largest insurance company in the world, namely Medicare, is not interested solely in cost. However, the contract for the work, issued by CMS, stipulated that the contractor could not publish study results without the approval of the US government.[5]

During the recent presidential campaign, both candidates stressed the importance of increased transparency in health care.[6,7] Both argued that increased information about quality and cost is essential to improving the US health care system. Almost all consumer groups want to know more about what works and what does not work and how quality varies by physician, hospital, or nursing home. Yet at least some of the research supported with public funds needed to produce this kind of information is to be performed under a process that allows the contracting agency to withhold results.

How should medicine respond to this situation? Even though the following recommendations may slow development of much needed quality measures, which in turn may slow progress in producing health care reform, they are important.

First, before physicians, or organizations comprising patients and physicians, agree to participate in a study about quality of care, they should ask whether the study directors are free to publish the results in a timely manner and whether the results will be submitted for peer review. If the answers to those questions is no, then physicians and organizations should refuse to participate in the study and should use the Internet and other means of mass communication to alert their professional networks about the situation.

Second, organizations such as the Joint Commission, the National Committee for Quality Assurance, and the National Quality Forum that either approve quality measures or use them for accreditation purposes should decline to use measures developed under a process that did not allow, at the time the work was conceptualized, for the work to be peer reviewed and published.

As health care reform is instituted in this political window, it will be difficult enough to convince the world that quality should be an equal partner with cost. It will be impossible if development of quality-related tools is clouded by lack of transparency. If the government is demanding transparency of physicians and hospitals, the very least the physicians and hospitals should do is demand transparency of the government.

A transparent process may still produce bad decisions, or result in publication of tools and the implementation of policies that in the long run produce more harm than good. But at least they will be developed using processes that reflect the value of a democratic society.

## References

1. CAL SB 680, § 898 October 14, 2001.

2. Carlisle D. *Access to Public Records Policy #02-5. 2002.* Memorandum to all Office of Statewide Health Planning and Development staff. http://www.oshpd.ca.gov/General_Info/PublicRecordsAct.pdf. November 17, 2008. Accessed August 15, 2008.

3. Office of Statewide Health Planning and Development. State of California public meetings Web page. http://www.oshpd.ca.gov/General_Info/Public_Meeting_Archive.html#CAP. Accessed August 15, 2008.

4. Centers for Medicare & Medicaid Services, Office of Acquisitions and Grant Management. Request for proposal No. RFP-CMS-MIDS-2008-0001. https://www.fbo.gov//utils/view?id=660d48ac12061672bae816e038d6dfce. May 2, 2008. Accessed March 6, 2008.

5. General Services Administration. *Rights in Data—Special Works.* Federal Acquisition Regulation §52.227-1 (December 2007).

6. Straight talk on health system reform. John McCain 2008. http://www.allhealth.org/BriefingMaterials/McCainPlan-1222.pdf. Accessed March 6, 2008.

7. Obama for America. Healthcare issues. http://www.barackobama.com/issues/healthcare. Accessed August 15, 2008.

# The Science of Health Care Reform

*Robert H. Brook, MD, ScD*
JAMA, *June 17, 2009—Vol. 301, No. 23, pp. 2486–2487*

Another health policy window has opened; through it will stream proposals to reform the US health care system. President Obama has demanded that reform proposals improve both coverage and quality of care and make health care more affordable for all Americans. Extending coverage without worrying about costs would be relatively easy. Improving quality of care without worrying about costs might also be achievable. But extending coverage and improving quality while also making coverage more affordable will be difficult.

The first step in pursuing the President's goals is to review what science has revealed about the system. Two studies could provide the context for health care reform. The first, the RAND Health Insurance Experiment (HIE),[1] was conducted more than 3 decades ago and would cost about 1 billion dollars to replicate today. The second, actually a combination of studies conducted mainly in the United States, is partially represented in the *Dartmouth Atlas*.[2]

The RAND HIE was a population- and community based, controlled experiment in which families from 6 sites across the country were randomized to 1 of 5 health insurance plans. There were 4 fee-for-service plans with different levels of cost sharing. Some families were randomized to free care in a health maintenance organization; their experiences were comparable with those of individuals in the fee-for-service system. The HIE's conclusions were straightforward: (1) increased cost sharing proportionally decreased health care use[1] and (2) on average, individuals with free care used about one-third more care than those in cost sharing plans, but at the end of 5 years, they were no healthier on average than their cost-sharing counterparts.[3]

The *Dartmouth Atlas* is the outcome of almost 3 decades of work examining use of health services in various geographic areas at a population level. The conclusions are straightforward: After controlling for demographic differences, health care use varies dramatically across both major geographic regions (as large as states) and smaller regions (such as hospital service areas), and at a population level, these large variations in health care do not translate into health differences.[4] Individuals living in regions of the country that use twice as much health care as other regions are not healthier.

The findings of these population-based studies seem to support policies that reduce service use in most geographic areas and increase what patients pay for care.

Such policies would not affect population-based health outcomes. However, from the perspective of an individual patient, the story is quite different.

In the HIE, the reason more care did not improve health is that providing more care did not improve the quality of care individuals received.[1] Furthermore, when patients had to pay for their own care, they reduced use of effective services in equal proportion to use of ineffective services.[1] These findings have been substantiated in more recent work.[5]

What does the individual patient perspective reveal about the *Dartmouth Atlas* findings? To answer this question, a series of studies in the 1990s examined the appropriateness of care in regions of the United States and the United Kingdom that had substantially different rates of overall use of health care services.[6–8] The studies found that perhaps one-third of common medical and surgical procedures are either equivocal (benefit and risk to the patient are about equal) or inappropriate (the procedure will produce more harm than benefit to that patient). Although this finding is disturbing, the relationship of appropriateness assessed at the individual patient level to health care services use in a given area is far more disquieting.

For instance, the use of coronary artery bypass graft (CABG) surgery in the 1980s in the Trent region of the United Kingdom was, on a population basis, one-seventh the use rate in southern California, where research had established that a substantial proportion of the procedures were performed for equivocal or inappropriate reasons. In the United Kingdom, where there was a National Health Service, regionalization, a small number of surgeons and cardiologists performing large volumes of procedures, and a use rate that was almost one seventh that of southern California, one might assume that all CABG surgeries would have been done for medically appropriate reasons. I attended cardiac case conferences in a major academic hospital in the Trent region and observed patients with severe left main coronary artery disease being placed on long waiting lists. However, a medical record review of patients who had undergone CABG surgery revealed that in about half the cases, the surgery was not appropriate.[8] Because these findings were so disquieting, the chief of cardiology at one of the hospitals individually reviewed every patient record and substantiated the findings.

On a population level, financial or supply constraints can be applied to control use, but some individuals will be harmed and some will benefit. As use rates in a geographic area increase, appropriateness remains about the same—some individuals will be harmed and some will benefit.[9]

Other studies have demonstrated the disconnect between variation in service use or policy changes on one hand and quality of care on the other. The only comprehensive national study of health care quality in the United States found that quality did not vary across geographic areas in which use of services varied dramatically.[10,11] In the HIE, quality of care was no better or individuals enrolled in the free plan than for those in cost sharing plans. The effect of Medicare's Prospective Payment System on quality of hospital care was generally a wash, even though the length of hospital stay decreased.[12] Care was somewhat better in the hospital, but some patients were discharged sicker and quicker, and those patients did not do well.[13]

How can physicians change the health care system in ways that both are sensitive to the needs of individual patients and reflect population-level data? Some suggestions follow.

First, however health care is reformed, the resulting system must explicitly assess the appropriateness of any major medical or surgical procedure before it is performed in a specific patient.

Second, the assessment of appropriateness must be based on reliable information. For example, previous work has shown that 40% of patients who had CABG surgery in New York State for left main coronary artery disease did not have the disease when coronary angiograms were read correctly.[14] Similarly, many appropriate surgery candidates were sent home without being offered CABG surgery because the angiograms were also inappropriately read.[14]

Third, the problems identified by the HIE and the *Dartmouth Atlas* need to be addressed by eliminating unnecessary care and wasted resources. Informal discussions with various specialists about the proportion of care they provide that does not meet their own definition of "necessary" suggests an amount ranging upward from 20%. If this is true, one way the President can begin to achieve his goals—without supply constraints or increased patient cost sharing—is by eliminating unnecessary care.

Fourth, it appears that simple interventions involving common clinical encounters may translate into large savings. For instance, most physicians order certain tests once a month, see patients once a year, and draw blood in the morning hours. What if physicians added 15% to a monthly or yearly interval and extended the frequency with which procedures are performed by 1 month or 1 year? This might produce a 1-time expenditure reduction that would help relieve some of the immediate pressure on the issue of affordability of health care. Perhaps in exchange for such changes, physicians could insist that health premiums be temporarily frozen for the population as a whole.

Fifth, perhaps it is time to address the affordability question head-on and insist that research about health care delivery focus on eliminating unnecessary care and wasted resources. There has been a substantial push to stimulate studies of comparative effectiveness. What criteria will be used to determine how federal money should be spent? What about a study only being conducted with taxpayer dollars on a new drug, device, or approach if it will replace something that is more expensive, guaranteeing up-front that what will be studied is less expensive? The study would have to determine whether what can be done less expensively will improve health or, at least, not harm patients.

What if industry used its own resources to fund independent evaluations of new drugs or devices that will be more expensive, regardless of their potential health effect? Changing the rules by which publicly funded comparative effectiveness studies are conducted might motivate the health care industry to refocus research and development on identifying drugs, devices, and tests that are better and less expensive rather than better and substantially more expensive.

Health care professionals need to help the President achieve the goals he has articulated. The goals cannot be achieved by controlling supply or increasing patient cost sharing. Such methods are too blunt when applied at an individual level: they will benefit some but harm others. It is time for physicians to commit as a profession to helping the President and Congress achieve the vision of a new health care system by improving the way medicine is practiced.

# References

1. Newhouse JP, Archibald RW, Bailit HL, et al. *Free for All? Lessons From the RAND Health Insurance Experiment.* Cambridge, MA: Harvard University Press; 1993.

2. Wennberg JE. *Tracking the Care of Patients With Severe Chronic Illness: The Dartmouth Atlas of Health Care 2008.* Lebanon, NH: Trustees of Dartmouth College; 2008.

3. Brook RH, Ware JE Jr, Rogers WH, et al. Does free care improve adults' health? results from a randomized controlled trial. *N Engl J Med.* 1983;309(23):1426-1434.

4. Skinner J, Chandra A, Goodman D, Fisher ES. The elusive connection between health care spending and quality. *Health Aff (Millwood).* 2009;28(1):w119-w123.

5. Goldman DP, Joyce GF, Escarce JJ, et al. Pharmacy benefits and the use of drugs by the chronically ill. *JAMA.* 2004;291(19):2344-2350.

6. Chassin MR, Kosecoff J, Park RE, et al. Does inappropriate use explain geographic variations in the use of health care services? a study of three procedures. *JAMA.* 1987;258(18):2533-2537.

7. Chassin MR, Kosecoff J, Park RE, et al, eds. *The Appropriateness of Use of Selected Medical and Surgical Procedures and Its Relationship to Geographic Variations in Their Use.* Ann Arbor, MI: Health Administration Press; 1989.

8. Gray D, Hampton JR, Bernstein SJ, Kosecoff J, Brook RH. Audit of coronary angiography and bypass surgery. *Lancet.* 1990;335(8701):1317-1320.

9. Park RE. Does inappropriate use explain small-area variations in the use of healthcare services—a reply. *Health Serv Res.* 1993;28(4):401-410.

10. McGlynn EA, Asch SM, Adams J, et al. The quality of health care delivered to adults in the United States. *N Engl J Med.* 2003;348(26):2635-2645.

11. Kerr EA, McGlynn EA, Adams J, Keesey J, Asch SM. Profiling the quality of care in twelve communities: results from the CQI study. *Health Aff (Millwood).* 2004;23(3):247-256.

12. Kahn KL, Rubenstein LV, Draper D, et al. The effects of the DRG-based prospective payment system on quality of care for hospitalized Medicare patients—an introduction to the series. *JAMA.* 1990;264(15):1953-1955.

13. Kosecoff J, Kahn KL, Rogers WH, et al. Prospective payment system and impairment at discharge—the quicker-and-sicker story revisited. *JAMA.* 1990;264(15):1980-1983.

14. Leape LL, Park RE, Bashore TM, Harrison JK, Davidson CJ, Brook RH. Effect of variability in the interpretation of coronary angiograms on the appropriateness of use of coronary revascularisation procedures. *Am Heart J.* 2000;139(1 pt 1):106-113.

# Possible Outcomes of Comparative Effectiveness Research

*Robert H. Brook, MD, ScD*
JAMA, *July 8, 2009—Vol. 302, No. 2, pp. 194–195*

With substantial support across the political spectrum, the Obama administration has included in the American Recovery and Reinvestment Act more than $1 billion to support comparative effectiveness research.[1] At the same time, the president has demanded reforms in the US health care system to make health care more affordable for all US citizens.[2] This Commentary focuses on the interaction of these 2 initiatives: what will be the cost effect of spending $1 billion on comparative effectiveness research?

First, it is important to understand what comparative effectiveness research will include. Discussions to date suggest that most of the funds will be spent comparing one clinical procedure, device, or drug with another.[3] The funds are less likely to be spent testing the comparative effectiveness of one way of paying for care vs another, of organizing care using a chronic disease model vs another organizational principle, or of implementing aggressive disease management programs.

Countless studies could be conducted to assess the comparative effectiveness of clinical procedures, devices, or drugs. Consider, for instance, a company that manufactures an improved surgical needle. Comparing that needle to the needle currently used could be included in comparative effectiveness research. A nearly infinite number of studies could be conducted to determine how often a person with back pain should receive chiropractic treatment, how often a patient with hypertension should receive follow-up care, how often a patient should obtain a dental checkup, or what form of radiation and chemotherapy will achieve the best outcome for a patient with cancer.

Since the government is using taxpayer dollars to fund the comparative effectiveness initiative, it would be appropriate to have an organizing principle to guide the selection of which aspects of medical care to examine. Without some overarching principle, the program is likely to become a free-for-all or a full employment program for health services researchers and epidemiologists. Researchers would submit proposals to study drug A vs B, or procedure A vs drug B. A study section would assess the proposals and decide which ones to fund, using the standard framework: the comparison should be important, the design should answer the question, and the study should be feasible to conduct.

But such an approach pays no attention to achieving the president's objective of making care more affordable or to insisting that the results of the comparative effectiveness studies be implemented quickly. So it is conceivable that most of the $1 billion could be allocated, for example, to testing a treatment that is more expensive than standard therapy to determine if the new treatment produces slightly better health. There is nothing wrong with such studies; the question is whether the scarce resources allocated in the stimulus package should be used in this way. It is clearly in the interest of companies that develop new treatments (eg, devices, drugs) to compare them with current or standard therapy. Why should taxpayer dollars subsidize that comparison and facilitate rapid entrance into the market of treatments that are slightly better but substantially more costly?

The comparative effectiveness funds should be allocated according to a framework designed to identify procedures, devices, and drugs that would reduce cost but not diminish health. This would help achieve the goal of making health care more affordable. Such a framework would have 2 new required features. First, a grant or contract to spend public money must include an initial analysis to establish a business case that implementing whatever is being proposed would reduce the cost of care by a certain percentage.

Second, it would not be enough to establish that implementing the new drug, device, or other therapy will save money. The history of science shows that it takes a long time for new knowledge to be incorporated into day-to-day practice.[4] So a second requirement for work funded under the stimulus package should be that successful innovations are implemented immediately. Thus, a successful application under the comparative effectiveness initiative must include constituents, such as health care organizations, hospitals, physicians, or organized community groups, that would agree to adopt the new therapy immediately if it were shown to be as safe as the old therapy but substantially less expensive. If such constituent letters were not contained in the grant proposal or contract under which the research would be conducted, the money should be spent investigating other topics.

Using comparative effectiveness funds correctly could foster a sea change in the way industry looks at product development. To return to the example of the new needle, the goal would no longer be to conduct a study to convince practitioners to pay more for a better needle. Rather, the goals would be to make better and safer needles, reduce the price of needles, and ensure that the new needles are adopted immediately. New radiation therapy machines would be required not only to produce the same level of health as the current ones but also to be substantially less expensive.

Showing the private sector that comparative effectiveness funds will be used in this way could change the entire research and development process in the US health care industry. It could also help the current administration achieve its goal of making health care more affordable for all US citizens.

To adopt these 2 criteria for funding comparative effectiveness research, the agencies that release funds must make tough decisions. The agencies will be accused of sponsoring rationing.[5] A strong case can be made that this does not represent rationing but rather uses research dollars to produce therapies that are better and substantially less expensive. After all, when a computer is purchased today at a small percentage of the cost of computers produced years ago, it is not believed that the private sector has rationed computer chips. Instead, the research and development model in the computer industry has been to make better machines and to make them at increasingly lower costs, thereby making computers affordable to many more individuals.

It is time to use public funding and comparative effectiveness research to accomplish the same thing in medicine. If this opportunity is missed, another one is unlikely to come along. Then rationing may actually become the only way by which reductions in health care expenditures can be achieved.

## References

1. The American Recovery and Reinvestment Act of 2009. US Government Printing Office Web site. http://frwebgate.access.gpo.gov/cgi-bin/getdoc.cgi?dbname=111_cong_bills&docid=f:h1enr.pdf. Accessibility verified June 10, 2009.

2. The White House. Issues: health care. http://www.whitehouse.gov/issues/health_care/. Accessed May 22, 2009.

3. Baucus M. *Call to Action Health Reform 2009.* Washington, DC: Senate Finance Committee; 2008.

4. McGlynn EA, Asch SM, Adams J, et al. The quality of health care delivered to adults in the United States. *N Engl J Med*. 2003;348(26):2635-2645.

5. Kyl J Senate Amendment 793 to Senate Continuing Resolution 13. 2009.

# Assessing the Appropriateness of Care—Its Time Has Come

*Robert H. Brook, MD, ScD*
JAMA, *September 2, 2009—Vol. 302, No. 9, pp. 997–998*

Health care reform in the United States is likely to fail without fundamental changes in the practice of medicine. What can be done within a year to substantially increase the likelihood that Americans receive appropriate, humane, affordable care? A starting point is to draw on more than 2 decades of empirical research based on the RAND/University of California Los Angeles (UCLA) Appropriateness Method (RUAM) to develop explicit criteria for determining the appropriateness of care.[1,2] Physicians and patients can use the results from applying this method to make better informed decisions about expensive, elective procedures or diagnostic tests, and the process of developing the criteria will strengthen the clinical evidence base.

The RUAM was developed more than 20 years ago in an effort to understand why quality of care in the United States, and in other developed countries, varied so substantially. The method uses a structured process for integrating findings from the scientific literature with clinical judgment to produce explicit criteria for determining the appropriateness of specific procedures.[1,2] The criteria are used to determine if care is necessary (the care produces substantially more health benefit than harm and is preferred over other available options), appropriate (produces more good than harm by a sufficiently wide margin to justify the use of the procedure), equivocal (potential health benefits and harms are about equal), or inappropriate (health risks are likely to exceed health benefits).

The RUAM has been used in research studies around the world, including England, Canada, Switzerland, the Netherlands, and Israel. This approach has been used to judge the appropriateness of a wide range of procedures, including bariatric surgery, coronary artery bypass graft surgery, angioplasty, colonoscopy, endoscopy, hysterectomy, prostatectomy, and tympanostomy, and has identified a large proportion of care as not necessary or appropriate (in some cases >50%).[3-9] The RUAM also has been used to identify underuse, patients for whom the procedure is necessary but to whom the procedure has not been offered by their physician.[10]

The goal of this work was not just to produce research results; it was intended to alter the way medicine is practiced. However, the only major nonresearch users became the insurance industry, which was looking for an evidence based method to review appropriateness, but having industry review appropriateness alienated physicians because they felt their clinical autonomy and judgment were threatened.

Times have changed and medical leaders are calling for greater accountability, especially in appropriateness of care. Using the existing appropriateness method as a foundation, the medical profession could begin guaranteeing Americans that an explicit assessment of appropriateness would be performed for at least 50 expensive, elective procedures or diagnostic tests, and that both patients and physicians would be an integral part of that process.

How might such a system work? The 50 sets of appropriateness criteria could be established on a national basis by 5 to 10 nonprofit organizations that have the requisite expertise, all using the RUAM. Doing this, and making associated improvements as the science of quality assessment evolves, would require about $100 million per year, most likely from federal sources. A coordinating center could ensure the consistency, quality, and timeliness of the work across these organizations. The initiative could also develop Web-accessible forms to produce appropriateness ratings for individual patients by following 8 steps: (1) select a procedure; (2) perform a literature review that includes information about use, efficacy, effectiveness, benefit, and risk for specific subgroups of patients; (3) develop an exhaustive and comprehensive set of clinical scenarios that describe both appropriate and inappropriate use of the procedure (scenarios may vary from <100 to >2000 per procedure); (4) select a multidisciplinary panel of 9 physicians to rate scenarios, after they read the literature review, on a scale of 1 to 9 (physicians who do not perform the procedure comprise a majority of the panel); (5) convene panel to discuss, modify, and rate the scenarios; (6) develop an efficient Web-based form that quickly but reliably allows the patient and physician to work together to determine the appropriateness score that is applicable to the specific patient; (7) use score to decide what to do next; and (8) continuously update literature review, clinical scenarios, and appropriateness ratings to keep them current with scientific progress.

Consider how an appropriateness assessment might work for a procedure such as carotid endarterectomy. Together, physician and patient would answer 12 to 15 questions on a Web-accessible form; the output would be an appropriateness score for this procedure for this specific patient. If the score was in the "necessary" or "appropriate" range, physician and patient might agree to proceed with the procedure, but there would be no requirement to do so. If the results were "equivocal" or "inappropriate," physician and patient might consider a different course of action.

Following the appropriateness assessment, physician and patient would indicate on the form whether they agreed with the assessment results. Clinical justification would be required if physician and patient decided to forego a necessary procedure or to have an equivocal or inappropriate procedure. Once the form was completed, it would become part of the patient's (hopefully) electronic medical record.

This explicit approach to appropriateness would dramatically change the current way of practicing medicine, and the drivers of change would be patients and physicians. Involving patients directly in an explicit assessment of appropriateness would increase their responsibility to understand what the appropriateness ratings mean and to engage in a more meaningful discussion with their physicians about their own care. This approach would also motivate physicians to document carefully the data used to make the appropriateness decision, thereby increasing the reliability of the process used to decide whether to order an expensive diagnostic test or therapeutic procedure.

A system for assessing appropriateness could be implemented quickly. By the end of a year, appropriateness criteria for at least 10 procedures could be available, and the system could be in use by physicians around the world. At the end of 2 years, the number of covered procedures could certainly be in the 20s, and in 3 years, 30 and so on. Because the way procedures would be selected for inclusion in the system would include total unit cost, frequency of use, and effects on patients' health, the proportion of health care dollars affected by the appropriateness system could be substantial.

The system needs to be supported by both professional and consumer organizations. Academic institutions should adopt the system to ensure that residents and interns understand how to provide appropriate and necessary care. The materials produced from the system could be used as teaching materials for both health professionals and consumer groups. The proportion of care delivered for appropriate or necessary reasons in an institution could be used to publicize individual training programs and increase transparency.

Use of this method could be mandated by organizations that accredit academic training programs; the Joint Commission could include it as part of its accreditation process. Professional societies involved in recertification could use data from the system to determine whether physicians who are being recertified provide appropriate and necessary care before they are allowed to sit for a recertification examination. Data from such a system could be used to stimulate research studies for procedures judged to be equivocal to produce a better clinical evidence base. Importantly, the performance of physicians, hospitals, or organizations would need to be audited on a sample basis to make sure that the appropriateness system was being properly used.

The appropriateness assessment system is a concrete way the medical profession could respond to the need to produce more efficient and effective care. Assessment can be performed in a manner consistent with both patient and physician values and allow for patient and physician autonomy; the assessment could also increase the reliability and validity of the clinical method. Implementing the system does not require the adoption of an information technology system or reorganization of the structure of medicine. If the RUAM is used as a starting point, a system can be operationalized within a year.

Unless specific action is taken to change the clinical process, 2 decades from now policy makers, physicians, health care organizations, and the public will still be discussing health care reform and debating vague approaches to making medicine in the United States and around the world more efficient and effective.

# References

1. Brook RH, Chassin MR, Fink A, Solomon DH, Kosecoff J, Park RE. A method for the detailed assessment of the appropriateness of medical technologies. *Int J Technol Assess Health Care.* 1986;2(1):53-63.

2. Fitch K, Bernstein S, Aguilar MS, Burnand B, et al. *The RAND/UCLA Appropriateness Method User's Manual 2001.* No. MR-1269-DG-XII/RE:126. Santa Monica, CA: RAND Corp; 2001.

3. Chassin MR, Kosecoff J, Park RE, et al. Does inappropriate use explain geographic variations in the use of health care services? a study of three procedures. *JAMA.* 1987;258(18):2533-2537.

4. Froehlich F, Burnand B, Pache I, et al. Overuse of upper gastrointestinal endoscopy in a country with open-access endoscopy: a prospective study in primary care. *Gastrointest Endosc.* 1997;45(1):13-19.

5. González N, Quintana JM, Lacalle JR, Chic S, Maroto D. Review of the utilization of the RAND appropriateness method in the biomedical literature (1999-2004). *Gac Sanit.* 2009;23(3):232-237.

6. Kleinman LC, Kosecoff J, Dubois RW, Brook RH. The medical appropriateness of tympanostomy tubes proposed for children younger than 16 years in the United States. *JAMA.* 1994;271(16):1250-1255.

7. Pilpel D, Fraser GM, Kosecoff J, Weitzman S, Brook RH. Regional differences in appropriateness of cholecystectomy in a prepaid health insurance system. *Public Health Rev.* 1992-1993;20(1-2):61-74.

8. Winslow CM, Solomon DH, Chassin MR, et al. The appropriateness of carotid endarterectomy. *N Engl J Med.* 1988;318(12):721-727.

9. Hemingway H, Chen R, Junghans C, et al. Appropriateness criteria for coronary angiography in angina. *Ann Intern Med.* 2008;149(4):221-231.

10. Kravitz RL, Laouri M, Kahan JP, et al. Validity of criteria used for detecting underuse of coronary revascularization. *JAMA.* 1995;274(8):632-638.

# Disruption and Innovation in Health Care

*Robert H. Brook, MD, ScD*
JAMA, *October 7, 2009—Vol. 302, No. 13, pp. 1465–1466*

Successful health care reform may provide virtually all individuals in the United States an adequate health insurance package. However, the need to increase value for health care dollars will extend far beyond the current policy window. Achieving that goal will require disruptive innovation in the health care system.

Disruption occurs when the expectations of individuals and the services provided are so vastly different that linear change is no longer likely.[1] For example, disruption occurred in naval warfare when reliance on battleships was replaced by aircraft carriers,[2] and in medicine when anesthesia and vaccines were introduced. Could similar kinds of successful disruption happen in the delivery of health care? There are 8 potential disruptions that could increase the value of health care.

First, the planet earth is no longer a stable environment, and its future, and that of the world's population, depends on how well it is treated. Therefore, it is reasonable to ask how changes in health care delivery would affect not just individuals, but the planet. A disruptive change would expand the view of health care policy beyond Congressional Budget Office scoring for cost and consider what proposed policies imply for the future of the planet. For example, how can the carbon footprint of new technologies and health facilities be reduced, and should new facilities be located in energy friendly places? How will increasing life expectancy affect the ability to reduce carbon dioxide emissions?

Second, improving delivery of health care services as they are now defined will do little to erase the difference in mortality and morbidity that exists in the United States as a function of where a person lives or who he or she is. Will the approach to health care delivery change to include at least some social determinants of health? Physicians do not spend sufficient time examining the social and mental health of patients, and do not view as their responsibility helping patients become better integrated into the community or developing positive mental health attributes that could make patients happier and, potentially, healthier.

Disruptive change could reach even further. What if the practice of pediatrics included examining the report cards of children or performing an independent assessment of a preschool child's readiness to read? What if a clinician explained to parents the importance of education and reading in being able to support a healthy lifestyle?

What if pay-for-performance included measures of educational attainment in addition to whether diabetes, hypertension, or asthma were controlled?

What would happen if the same fundamental disruption occurred in the school system so that teachers were responsible not only for the educational achievement of students, but also for their health? Would there be more willingness to spend education dollars to reduce posttraumatic stress and depression in children so they were ready to learn? Until now, education and medical care have operated in 2 silos. Will there be a disruption that at least brings these 2 great social systems together to integrate some aspects of the social determinants of health with the delivery of personal medical services?

Third, society has made substantial efforts to protect individuals against health practitioners who may do more harm than good or are not qualified to treat a given condition or a specific patient. Traditionally educated but independent nurse practitioners with physician backup can produce, for selected patients, a comparable level of care as physicians.[3] Likewise, women with low-risk pregnancies managed during delivery by midwives with physician backup vs those managed in a consultant-led labor had fewer interventions without differences in fetal outcomes.[4] Will the system be disrupted by allowing and fostering the development of educational models that base acceptance on whether a clinician can do something as opposed to how that clinician is educated and trained?

The health services research literature is replete with information about the volume-outcome relationship; for selected procedures, doing something more produces better results. If the sole focus of a clinician is removing cataracts, performing colonoscopies, injecting Botox, or reading mammograms, why can't individuals be trained to perform these activities without requiring them to graduate from medical school? Perhaps a new approach to training should be considered that combines skills from nursing, public health, and medicine.[5] Perhaps high school graduates with appropriate physician supervision could perform some tasks that currently only physicians are legally permitted to perform.

Fourth, substantial resources are invested in building places to provide health care services or acquiring new equipment. Will there be an attempt to disrupt the way medicine is currently practiced and make it a 24-hour business so that routine office visits, nonemergency tests, including magnetic resonance imaging, outpatient surgeries, and vaccinations are available around the clock? If so, will incentives be offered to individuals who use facilities at off-peak hours? Would making health care a 24-hour business protect the planet while driving down the cost of medical care because capital will not be needed to build new buildings and purchase new equipment to replace buildings and equipment that had many more uses left in their lifespan?

Fifth, can the culture of medicine be dramatically changed to root out waste? Almost every other business is determined to make better products for less money.

Will waste reduction be made a central focus so that the practice of medicine changes dramatically?[6,7]

Sixth, will there be a commitment to a globalized health care delivery system, thereby perhaps eliminating jobs in one country and generating them in another? For instance, elective surgery could be performed with high quality and less cost outside the United States,[8] and x-rays could be read instantaneously by radiologists located in another country. Instead, will medicine continue to be practiced on a statewide or countrywide basis?

Seventh, will professional associations commit to being responsible for both cost and quality on a population basis and will board certification depend on performance in both dimensions? Shouldn't the highlight of any national meeting of any group of health professionals be a presentation describing how the value of health care dollars has been increased in the last year and how health and cost have been addressed simultaneously on a population basis?

Eighth, what are the rights and responsibilities of both patients and physicians? Does a clinician have a responsibility to advise a patient to stop smoking or to get a mammogram? Does the responsibility include sending a reminder for a mammography appointment, or scheduling an appointment at a time convenient for the patient?

Moreover, what is the patient's responsibility? For example, if a patient who does not receive a colonoscopy (even though the procedure is covered by insurance and scheduled at a convenient time) develops colon cancer, does that patient have the right to expect the same services that would be provided for a patient who developed colon cancer but had received a colonoscopy?

None of the potential disruptions described in this article will affect the current political window for policy change in the United States. But they need to be on the agenda for discussion so a better health care system can be built for the future.

Currently, legislators considering whether to build more medical schools look at what physicians do, determine how the population is changing, multiply those 2 factors, and compare the product with the denominator of physician work hours that would be available without expanding medical schools. The result is usually a decision to build new medical schools. But if disruptive changes in the training of health professionals are possible, the need for more physicians could be altered dramatically, and perhaps resources allocated for more medical schools could be conserved and spent on more valuable activities. For instance, some of the money should be invested to produce a new science of health care delivery that investigates changes in the practice of medicine that would be labeled disruptive. Otherwise scientific studies on health care delivery will produce, at best, changes at the margin that will have little effect on cost, quality, or health.

# References

1. Bower JL, Christensen CM. Disruptive technologies—catching the wave. *Harv Bus Rev.* 1995;73(1):43-53.

2. Hundley RO; US Defense Advanced Research Projects Agency; National Defense Research Institute; RAND Corporation. *Past Revolutions, Future Transformations: What Can the History of Revolutions in Military Affairs Tell Us About Transforming the US Military?* Santa Monica, CA: RAND Corporation; 1999.

3. Mundinger MO, Kane RL, Lenz ER, et al. Primary care outcomes in patients treated by nurse practitioners or physicians: a randomized trial. *JAMA.* 2000; 283(1):59-68.

4. Hundley VA, Cruickshank FM, Lang GD, et al. Midwife managed delivery unit—a randomized controlled comparison with consultant-led care. *BMJ.* 1994;309 (6966):1400-1404.

5. Mundinger MO, Starck P, Hathaway D, Shaver J, Woods NF. The ABCs of the doctor of nursing practice: assessing resources, building a culture of clinical scholarship, curricular models. *J Prof Nurs.* 2009;25(2):69-74.

6. New England Health Care Institute. *How Many More Studies Will It Take? A Collection of Evidence That Our Health Care System Can Do Better.* Cambridge, MA: New England Health Care Institute; 2008.

7. Bentley TG, Effros RM, Palar K, Keeler EB. Waste in the US health care system: a conceptual framework. *Milbank Q.* 2008;86(4):629-659.

8. Milstein A, Smith M. Will the surgical world become flat? *Health Aff (Millwood).* 2007;26(1):137-141.

# Continuing Medical Education: Let the Guessing Begin

*Robert H. Brook, MD, ScD*
JAMA, *January 27, 2010—Vol. 303, No. 4, pp. 359–360*

Patients expect their physicians to have the right answer every time. Does the testing process in medical school or the continuing medical education (CME) process increase the likelihood that patient expectations will be met?

A medical student finishing Step 1 or Step 2 examinations receives a score. The score reflects answers that the student knew, answers chosen by process of elimination, or answers the student guessed correctly. The Medical Knowledge Self-Assessment Program[1] is an authoritative manual designed to update internists on the practice of medicine over the previous 3 years. Each section of the document ends with a series of multiple-choice questions. The physician selects responses and submits the answers to the American College of Physicians, which awards the CME credits.

How should the medical student or the practicing physician feel about answering 70% of the questions correctly? Is the testing system at the heart of why quality-of-care scores for individual practices are so low?[2]

The purpose of this Commentary is to suggest exploration of a culture shift in medicine to reinforce the notion of knowing the right answer every time.

What if the testing process in medical school or CME were changed so that the medical student or physician were faced with a problem and had to decide what to do? This experience would teach a physician how to look up information, read articles, determine if the articles were relevant, and how to apply the literature and evidence-based medicine to individual patients.

Such an approach raises concern if a physician needs to know immediately what to do. So what if a list of medical emergencies and related patient scenarios was developed, as well as a system for reminding all physicians, regardless of specialty, what to do in these situations? Certain types of chest pain, headaches, and other symptoms would fall in this category. In these cases, physicians should know the correct answer 100% of the time without looking it up. For the rest of medical practice, shouldn't physicians be taught how to find the answer and be confident that it is correct?

To accomplish the latter, evidence-based medicine must be translated into practice. Although the movement for evidence-based medicine began nearly 2 decades ago,[3] little progress has been made in adopting the tools of evidence-based medicine into routine practice. Systematic reviews grade and synthesize evidence from diverse studies and many of these meta-analyses are used. But there is little documentation about how they have been used and whether they have affected practice. Beyond that, what about the simplest tools of quantitative sciences? Are the concepts of prior probability, posterior probability, transforming a prior probability into a posterior probability, or any other principles in decision analysis used in medicine?

After reading the first half of the Medical Knowledge Self-Assessment Program curriculum for internists, I was fascinated by the absence of any quantitative decision tools. The field of decision analysis has produced numerous studies about using decision tools to improve the practice of medicine. Dean et al[4] demonstrated that a decision tool could ensure that a patient received the correct antibiotic. Years ago Adams et al[5] demonstrated how a simple decision tool could help to decide whether a patient who presents to an emergency department with abdominal pain needs surgery.

Private firms are beginning to collect decision tools and make them available to physicians. However, in general, use of sensitivity, specificity, likelihood ratios, prior probabilities, and posterior probabilities in medical decision making has been largely ignored. An entire field of science is missing from the practice of medicine. At the same time, production of a slightly better drug or device prompts a full scale advertising campaign, backed by a sales force.

Despite almost 800 reports on the Framingham risk score[6] this decade, few physicians enter on a patient's record the probability that the patient will have a cardiac event in the next 10 years. Why are there no formal assessments of probabilities and utilities in making difficult clinical decisions? When a patient enters a physician's office, why doesn't the physician record a prior probability that the patient has condition x, y, or z; then, based on the history and physical, produce a posterior probability that serves as the basis for ordering tests?

Thirty years ago, a physician had to know what laboratory tests to order. He or she might have been required to write the test legibly on a laboratory order slip. With today's electronic medical record–supported process, the physician views a computer screen that provides a long list of tests, organized by organ system, or in some other way. The physician can indicate which test to order without knowing the purpose for which the test was designed—is it specific, sensitive, neither—and without knowing the cost of performing it.

A physician cannot remember all of the tests and resulting decisions that must be made but the situation is going to explode exponentially over the next 5 to 10 years as a multitude of new tests come to market to measure specific aspects of a patient's genetic, proteinic, or physiological nature. Facing such complexity, will this result in incorporating validated rules and tools into the practice of medicine so that physicians can make the right diagnosis, and monitor therapy, at a price that society is willing to pay?

At the Johns Hopkins Medical School 30 years ago, one of the most popular lectures given dealt with the diagnosis of syphilis. The professor who gave the lecture handed out his business card. The back of the card displayed an algorithm that showed how to treat the patient depending on whether a test result was positive or negative, or whether the test was performed on spinal fluid or blood. The card also indicated when students needed to call the professor because test results were inconsistent. It was one of the few business cards that house officers kept.

Thirty years later, scant progress has been made in applying evidence-based decision tools to practice. Physicians should know they can get the correct answer all of the time because they know how to arrive at the answer; and they must understand which emergency situations require them to know what to do instantly. Decision making in medicine will be more valid and reliable by incorporating the sciences of decision analysis and clinical evidence into the routine practice of medicine.

With few exceptions, physicians are using the same information sciences that were used 30 years ago. It is time for a change before innovative medical researchers develop a new array of tests and measurements, making it even less likely that physicians will have the right answer.

## References

1. Alguire PC, Epstein PE; American College of Physicians. *MKSAP 14: Medical Knowledge Self-Assessment Program*. Philadelphia, PA: American College of Physicians; 2006.

2. McGlynn EA, Asch SM, Adams J, et al. The quality of health care delivered to adults in the United States. *N Engl J Med*. 2003;348(26):2635-2645.

3. Sackett DL. *Clinical Epidemiology: A Basic Science for Clinical Medicine*. Boston, MA: Little Brown; 1985.

4. Dean NC, Silver MP, Bateman KA, James B, Hadlock CJ, Hale D. Decreased mortality after implementation of a treatment guideline for community-acquired pneumonia. *Am J Med*. 2001;110(6):451-457.

5. Adams ID, Chan M, Clifford PC, et al. Computer aided diagnosis of acute abdominal pain: a multicentre study. *Br Med J (Clin Res Ed)*. 1986;293(6550): 800-804.

6. Bibliography for Framingham Heart Study. http://www.framinghamheartstudy.org/biblio/index.html. Accessed December 18, 2009.

# The Primary Care Physician and Health Care Reform

*Robert H. Brook, MD, ScD (RAND Corporation)*
*Roy T. Young, MD (Eisenhower Medical Center, Rancho Mirage, California)*
*JAMA, April 21, 2010—Vol. 303, No. 15, pp. 1535–1536*

Whatever form it takes, Health Care Reform will increase the number of Americans covered by health insurance. But there is concern that the legislation will not bend the cost curve—that is, will not reduce the growth of health care costs so that it more closely resembles the growth of the US gross domestic product (GDP). Currently, health care consumes about 16% of the GDP; advocates of bending the cost curve hope that in 2020 it will still consume roughly the same proportion.

Increased health care coverage raises issues in addition to cost containment. Increased coverage will mean increased demand for primary care physicians. Virtually everyone would like to have a primary care physician—a trusted physician who provides comprehensive, continuous care. Many studies, including many with international comparisons, have established the benefits of primary care.[1] However, it is increasingly difficult to convince graduates of US medical schools to choose primary care as their professional career path. Why is there such a disconnect between the demand for and supply of primary care physicians? Two reasons appear to predominate: scope of practice and salary.

## Scope of Practice

The scope of practice for primary care physicians is contracting. There are 900 million visits to physicians annually in the United States,[2] and about half of these are to the 200,000 physicians who identified themselves as office based primary care clinicians.[3] These physicians manage most of the care for diabetes, hypertension, and obesity; address acute problems such as viral or bacterial infections; and provide general examinations. On the other hand, a large proportion of the visits for conditions that could be managed by primary care physicians such as rheumatoid arthritis, epilepsy, depression, angina pectoris, and other chronic conditions are diagnosed and managed over time by specialists.[2] The role of primary care physicians in the hospital has also narrowed, driven by the emergence of hospitalists and the trend to move a substantial portion of medical care to outpatient facilities.

## Salary

The salary differential between a primary care physician and a specialist is substantial. The median salary in large, multispecialty group practice for a US internist is about $205,000 a year; for a family medicine physician, $198,000; and for a pediatrician, $203,000. The median dermatologist salary is $351,000.[4] Given this pay differential and the narrowed scope of practice, why should bright, hardworking, debt-ridden, or even altruistic medical students choose internal medicine, family medicine, pediatrics, or primary care for residency?

In 2010, only 2722 (54.5%) of the 4999 residency spots in internal medicine were filled by graduates of US-based allopathic medical schools; respective numbers for family medicine residency were 1169 (44.8%) of 2608, and for pediatrics, 1711 (70.5%) of 2428.[5] In comparison, at least 90% of positions in neurological surgery, orthopedic surgery, and dermatology were filled by US medical school graduates.[5] Young clinicians are simply not willing to forfeit lifetime earnings of over $3 million even though the medicine they would practice as primary care physicians is critical to improving the health of patients and to making the current health system more functional.[6] To many of these students, the primary care physician might seem a lot like the water boy on a football team making sure that the really important members of the medical team do their work.

Many reports have lamented the current situation. For example, the Society of General Internal Medicine (SGIM) published a report enthusiastically defining the roles of a primary care physician and arguing why these roles are so important to the health care system.[7] The American Academy of Family Physicians (AAFP) Statement Report reconfirms the worsening shortage of primary care physicians.[8] Many efforts are underway to enhance the environment in which primary care physicians practice, including building medical homes, developing accountable health care organizations, and installing information technology systems. All of these initiatives could substantially improve the lives of primary care physicians, making it more intellectually stimulating, as well as feasible and efficient to provide integrated, continuous care.[9] But despite efforts to highlight the potential clinical and professional contributions of primary care physicians, interest in this path remains extraordinarily low among graduates of US medical schools.

## A Possible Solution

One approach to this situation is to do nothing. As a result, the number of primary care physicians in practice will continue to decline. Patients who want a primary care physician will probably need to pay some kind of retainer and enroll in a concierge-type practice. Those who cannot afford this luxury will have to endure a medical care system that is even more fragmented than it is today.

An alternative approach is to convince 50% of students entering US medical schools, starting in June 2010, to choose primary care (pediatrics, family medicine, or general internal medicine) as their professional career path. The suggestions of multiple task forces for making delivery of primary care easier can be implemented. For this approach to be successful, a way must be found to reduce the pay differential between primary care physicians and specialists.

In addition to fulfilling the roles so eloquently outlined by the SGIM[7] and AAFP[8] taskforces, primary care physicians must lead the effort to bend the cost curve and eliminate variations in health care expenditures based solely on where one lives rather than on medical need. If successful, a Dartmouth Atlas produced in 2020 would confirm that variation in expenditures on health care is related to need, not to geography.[10]

To achieve these goals, primary care physicians need a different set of clinical responsibilities and skills. They must become leaders in efforts to avoid preventable hospitalizations for patients with chronic diseases, eliminate inappropriate or equivocal surgery and radiologic procedures, and help individuals die with the least pain and without expenditures of vast amounts of money. The workflow of the medical system must be redesigned so that primary care clinicians can perform procedures and carry out tasks for which they have been trained. In addition, for patients with single or multiple chronic illnesses, primary care physicians must provide a greater proportion of the continuing care.[2]

The contract primary care physicians must make with the public is simple: If society working with insurance companies, Medicare, and Medicaid would close the salary gap between primary care physicians and specialists, primary care physicians would lead the medical profession in eliminating unnecessary variations in care and bending the cost curve, in addition to being the trusted allies of patients by providing high-quality care. Will expanding the scope of practice and increasing salaries motivate enough medical students to forsake careers in higher paying specialties? Or will the fascination of working at the cutting edge of medical technology still capture the minds and hearts of most medical students? The answer is unknown; however, it is certain that if the salary gap cannot be closed and the role of the primary care physician redefined in a powerful way, there is little hope of producing a health care system that provides high-quality affordable care to the US population.

## References

1. Starfield B, Shi LY, Macinko J. Contribution of primary care to health systems and health. *Milbank Q.* 2005;83(3):457-502.

2. Cherry DK, Hing E, Woodwell DA, Rechtsteiner EA. *National Ambulatory Medical Care Survey: 2006 Summary.* Vol 3. Hyattsville, MD: Centers for Disease Control and Prevention, National Center for Health Statistics; 2008.

3. American Medical Association. *Physician Characteristics and Distribution in the U.S.* Chicago, IL: Survey & Data Resources, American Medical Association; 2009.

4. *Medical Group Compensation & Financial Survey.* Alexandria, Va: American Medical Group Association; 2009.

5. More US medical school seniors to train as family medicine residents. *medicalnewstoday.com.* March 19, 2010. http://www.medicalnewstoday.com/articles/182874.php. Accessed March 22, 2010.

6. Steinbrook R. Easing the shortage in adult primary care—is it all about money? *N Engl J Med.* 2009;360(26):2696-2699.

7. Larson EB, Fihn SD, Kirk LM, et al; Task Force on the Domain of General Internal Medicine. Society of General Internal Medicine (SGIM). The future of general internal medicine: report and recommendations from the Society of General Internal Medicine (SGIM) Task Force on the Domain of General Internal Medicine. *J Gen Intern Med.* 2004;19(1):69-77.

8. Statement AAFP: recruitment report reconfirms worsening shortage of primary care physicians [news release]. Leawood, KS: American Academy of Family Physicians; June 25, 2009. http://www.aafp.org/online/en/home/media/releases /newsreleases-statements-2009/merritthawkins-physicianshortage.html. Accessed March 22, 2010.

9. Rittenhouse DR, Shortell SM, Fisher ES. Primary care and accountable care—two essential elements of delivery-system reform. *N Engl J Med.* 2009;361(24):2301-2303.

10. Wennberg JE, Fisher EG, Goodman DC, Skinner JS. *Tracking the Care of Patients with Severe Chronic Illness—The Dartmouth Atlas of Health Care 2008.* New Hampshire, Lebanon: Dartmouth Medical School; 2008.

# Rights and Responsibilities in Health Care: Striking a Balance

*Robert H. Brook, MD, ScD*
JAMA, *June 9, 2010—Vol. 303, No. 22, pp. 2289–2290*

In many states, teenagers can apply for a driver's license when they are 16 years old. To obtain the license, they need to pass a written examination, perform adequately on a driving test, and demonstrate that they have insurance. But all drivers can do things to lose their license. For example, the law requires that drivers stop at red lights, even in the middle of the night when the street is empty. If drivers choose to ignore this law, they risk being ticketed; enough tickets will probably cost them the right to drive. These requirements are not arbitrary; they were developed to preserve life and reduce the cost of everyone's insurance.

When young adults are 26 years old, they can no longer be covered under their parents' health insurance plan. However, they have other coverage options. If they work, and their employer offers insurance, they need only check a box. If they apply for an individual policy, they may need to prove that they do not have preexisting conditions and will need to provide extensive background information. But in either case, they do not need to know about the health care system or how to use it efficiently and appropriately. Misuse of the system may cost them a monetary penalty, but for these young adults, those penalties will seem far less important compared with the loss of their license to drive.

What if this approach to health insurance changed? What if to obtain and keep health insurance, individuals had to pass something like a driver's license test? What should they study to prepare for the test? What should be taught? What skills should be demonstrated? Should insurance be more costly, or even withdrawn, not because individuals become sick but because they do not use preventive services or evidence-based care in a manner that both protects their health and reduces health care costs for others? If society both provides health insurance and helps those who do not have the ability to use services effectively, what kind of penalty for misuse would be ethically and morally acceptable? Should penalties and rewards be applied first to the middle class, as opposed to disadvantaged individuals who are enrolled in Medicaid?[1]

Over the last 40 years, tests and drugs have been developed that can predict or change the course of illness—even a potentially silent condition such as hypertension. The medical profession has responded to these changes by teaching physicians skills for motivating patients to obtain necessary diagnostic tests, take necessary medications, be vaccinated, and receive routine preventive services. However, physicians have not had remarkable success in improving adherence to necessary interventions, such as those for hypertension,[2] or in containing the costs of providing care. Is it time to admit that unless patients assume greater responsibility, these problems will not be solved?

For instance, consider a health system in which individuals who have health insurance and are competent to care for themselves would be required to take medications and have procedures known to be necessary and would do so; and a severe penalty would be imposed if they do not. What if individuals were required to receive vaccines for which they were eligible, as soon as the vaccines became available—and were penalized if they contracted an illness the vaccination could have prevented?

What if individuals with hypertension or hyperlipidemia who did not take their medications became responsible for some of the costs of future cardiac care? If the nation's future health system is expected to contain costs and improve value, shouldn't the recipients be expected to be true partners in achieving those goals?

This kind of sea change would take time to implement, would need to be preceded by education, and should be first implemented among individuals for whom language or competence would not be a barrier to getting required care. This policy would also need to focus on medications and procedures for which effectiveness has been well established.

Blue ribbons and awards are given to health plans for having high mammogram rates, high colonoscopy rates, and appropriate levels of hemoglobin A1c and low-density lipoprotein cholesterol among their members.[3] Perhaps the awards should be given to patients instead of physicians and health organizations. Perhaps it is time to say to the American public: "Certain procedures, medications, and preventive care will make a difference in your health, and it is your responsibility, not your physician's, to take or to do them."

If individuals want to use their car warranty to get repairs, they have to show that they have provided at least minimal maintenance. In general, individuals agree that minimal maintenance is a fair trade-off for using a warranty. What is the fair trade-off in medical care? If patients do not take prescribed medications, are not appropriately vaccinated, or do not obtain preventive screening tests, they may incur costs that others will need to subsidize. Is that fair?

Moreover, behaviors like smoking, use of illicit drugs, alcoholism, and dietary patterns leading to obesity greatly contribute to both poor health and increased medical expenditures.[4] Although individuals are responsible for these behaviors, their prevalence is determined by many factors, most of them not under an individual's control.[5,6] Nevertheless, there are ways to begin increasing patient responsibility for these problems. Should parents be expected to maintain their young children's weight-to-height index at the 50th percentile or less? Should sedentary workers be expected to participate in an exercise program provided at the workplace?

Classes using sophisticated adult learning materials could be held in the workplace. Employees could choose which health plan to join—one that required them to use the health care system responsibly, or one that did not—with the understanding that the former would be less expensive. Premium savings from using health services responsibly could be returned to the worker as a bonus. Such initiatives are already being implemented by progressive employers.[7] To have an even greater effect, these initiatives would need to be widely adopted, and governmental support would be needed to pursue penalties and awards more aggressively.

Health reform is not only about health insurance companies, physicians, and pharmaceutical and device companies. It is not only mandating health insurance for everyone. It is not only about subsidies and penalties for not buying insurance.[8,9] Health reform is about people. And people must become full participants and assume much greater responsibility for their actions if health benefits are to be maintained at an affordable cost.

The health reform bill signed by President Obama includes funding for numerous demonstration projects. Perhaps a demonstration project that contains some of the elements discussed herein will be tried, evaluated, and result in a new approach to the delivery of health care. Responsible patients and responsible communities might make it easier for physicians to act responsibly and to increase their effectiveness and cost-effectiveness. Maybe then, everyone would be able to purchase a health plan that provides necessary, high-quality, humane, and affordable care; by doing so, the health of individuals and the health of the nation would improve.

## References

1. Steinbrook R. Imposing personal responsibility for health. *N Engl J Med*. 2006;355(8):753-756.

2. Institute of Medicine. *A Population-Based Policy and Systems Change Approach to Prevent and Control Hypertension*. Washington, DC: Institute of Medicine; 2010.

3. Comarow A. America's best health insurance plans. *US News World Rep*. 2009;146(11):91.

4. Goldman DP, Zheng Y, Girosi F, et al. The benefits of risk factor prevention in Americans aged 51 years and older. *Am J Public Health*. 2009;99(11):2096-2101.

5. Marmot M. *Fair Society, Healthy Lives—The Marmot Review: Strategic Review of Health Inequalities in England Post 2010*. London, England: Marmot Review; 2010.

6. Cohen DA. Neurophysiological pathways to obesity: below awareness and beyond individual control. *Diabetes*. 2008;57(7):1768-1773.

7. Linnan L, Bowling M, Childress J, et al. Results of the 2004 National Worksite Health Promotion Survey. *Am J Public Health*. 2008;98(8):1503-1509.

8. Affordable Health Care for America Act, HR 3962, 111th Cong, 1st Sess (2009).

9. Patient Protection and Affordable Care Act, Pub L No. 111-148, 124 Stat 119 (2010).

# Medical Leadership in an Increasingly Complex World

*Robert H. Brook, MD, ScD*
JAMA, *July 28, 2010—Vol. 304, No. 4, pp. 465–466*

Greece is going bankrupt. The Euro is shaky. The oil inundating the Gulf Coast may eliminate one-third of the US seafood catch. In the midst of this chaos, the nightly news focuses on a medical breakthrough. At a cost of about $100,000, a man with metastatic prostate cancer can be treated with an infusion of his own cells and live, on average, a few months longer.[1] The commentator questions whether insurance companies will pay for this therapy and wonders whether men who do not have metastatic cancer will demand access to the therapy, even if they have to pay for it themselves. Perhaps Yeats was right—"Things fall apart; the centre cannot hold."[2]

The United States spends more money per person on medical care than any other developed country in the world. But Americans are not the healthier for it.[3] Life expectancy in the United States is lower than in virtually any other developed country, and variation in life expectancy, as a function of where a person lives or grows up, is high. In the context of this dismal reality, consider the assertion in the Declaration of Independence that every citizen has the right to life, liberty, and the pursuit of happiness. What should be expected from a physician leader in this complex world?

Physicians are found in leadership positions throughout US society but are rarely at the top. Physicians have been elected to both houses of Congress, but no physician has been elected president. Medical leaders are found in the executive branch of the Department of Health and Human Services, but virtually never at its highest levels.

But physicians have extraordinary influence. They run the programs that spend large amounts of money to treat the elderly and the poor, at both state and national levels. They provide a moral compass when they serve as surgeon general. And most frequently, they are responsible for running large health care delivery systems and for training the future health workforce of the United States.

Indeed, the teaching role has expanded from being a dean of a medical school to overseeing the entire health enterprise of an academic campus, including teaching hospitals and schools of medicine, nursing, pharmacy, and public health. Physicians also control all of the organizations that set professional standards in medicine, from individual specialty societies to organizations cutting across the entire medical establishment.

What defines a successful leader of such organizations? That's more than a rhetorical question. Medicine now makes up 17% of the US gross domestic product; thus, a large part of the country's ability to ensure life, liberty, and the pursuit of happiness is in the hands of medical leaders.

There are several possible definitions of successful leadership. Is it an indication of success if the leader of an academic medical center keeps the institution financially solvent, constructs new buildings—especially those for basic science research—moves the institution higher on the National Institutes of Health grant list, and trains physicians to concentrate on the patient by using all tools at their disposal? Are leaders of professional societies successful when they persuade Congress that the society's members provide great scientific value and thus merit higher salaries; or if those leaders convince philanthropies to donate a disproportionate amount of money to that specialty? Is the leader of a major program, such as Medicare, successful when bills are paid promptly, adequate reimbursement is made for services rendered, and services are provided with high quality and little waste? Is the medical leader of a pharmaceutical company successful when the company develops a product that increases life expectancy by 3 months at a price of $100,000 and then convinces the public and insurers that patients must have the product and that it must be paid for with public money?

Many would answer yes in all of these cases. Who wants a leader of an academic medical center who builds nothing, does not attract research grants, and fails to maintain financial stability? Certainly not the center's board of governance. But in this complex world, are these sufficiently inclusive definitions of a successful physician leader?

There are 3 competing models for improving health in a population. The first, for which virtually all of the resources are used, is the medical model, in which an individual patient visits a physician who uses his or her clinical training to diagnose and treat the patient. The second is the public health model, driven primarily by the quest to eliminate root causes of population behavior that produces poor health, such as drug addiction, obesity, alcoholism, and cigarette smoking. The third, a more recent force, is the social determinants of health model,[4] which argues that neither the medical nor public health model is sufficient to improve the health of a population. Rather, improving health may require a wide range of strategies, including redistribution of wealth; guaranteeing all adults access to a meaningful job that pays an income sufficient to allow them to pursue healthy behaviors; helping children feel safe and be healthy and ready to learn; and empowering women and communities so that they can work more effectively to increase the health of the population.

All 3 models must be pursued in balance. All medical leaders, no matter what their position, should be prepared to answer the following questions. What have I done to improve the health of the US population, or my entire community, and how did I take advantage of all 3 frameworks that produce health most efficiently? If I am trying to improve the health of a community, how do I balance investment in the social determinants of health, a classical public health approach, and more medical care? How do

I develop a plan for my specialty society, my medical group, and my academic medical center that will help make them not only advocates for a better personal health care system but also advocates for better health?

What if vice chancellors, provosts, and medical leaders were required to produce an annual report describing how they improved the health of the community in which the academic facility existed? What if leaders of professional societies were asked similar questions? What if medical students, nursing students, public health students, and students of economics, anthropology, and sociology were required to find ways to work together to improve health?

What if during their medical school interview, bright college students challenged their interviewers to explain what the school does to help the community and how the school's activities encompass the priorities of a better health care delivery system, better public health, and the social determinants of health? What if before joining a specialty society, physicians inquired about the society's plan for improving health in a manner that the United States can afford and asked if the society's meetings would include presentations by individuals who have other than a medical background?

Long ago, the United States articulated common values of achievement for citizens. However, in the pursuit of building institutions, physicians have paid too little attention to the common values specified in the nation's founding documents. Moving a society toward health is difficult. But perhaps it is time to expand the notion of medical leadership and demand that leaders be accountable for explaining how their leadership is focused on improving health, reducing its variation, and doing so in an affordable way.

Many of the best and the brightest students still choose medicine as a career, and the medical establishment is justly proud of its achievements. But the world has moved on. It is time for physicians to think beyond making their institution, practice, or professional society better. The population needs, and deserves, such leadership. And physicians can provide it.

## References

1. Bazelle R. New prostate cancer treatment explained. http://www.msnbc.msn.com/id/34276015/vp/36871290#36871290. Accessed June 15, 2010.

2. Yeats WB. The Second Coming. In: *Michael Robartes and the Dancer*. Cruchtown, Ireland: The Chuala Press; 1920.

3. *OECD Health Data 2009 Statistics and Indicators for 30 Countries*. 18th ed. Paris, France: Institut de Recherche et Documentation en Economie de la Santé; 2009.

4. Marmot M. Closing the health gap in a generation: the work of the Commission on Social Determinants of Health and its recommendations. *Glob Health Promot*. 2009(suppl 1):23-27.

# Physician Compensation, Cost, and Quality

*Robert H. Brook, MD, ScD*
JAMA, *August 18, 2010—Vol. 304, No. 7, pp. 795–796*

Traditionally, there have been 3 ways to reimburse physicians for services rendered: salary, capitation, or fee for service. A physician who receives a salary is paid a certain amount per month or year of work. Physicians reimbursed through capitation are paid based on the number of patients they see or the number of patients for whom they are responsible. Physicians reimbursed on a fee-for-service basis are paid for every service they provide, regardless how simple or complex.

The way physicians are paid affects, even if subconsciously, what physicians do. If salaried physicians believe that spending hours on a well-child or routine adult health maintenance visit is clinically desirable and there are no administrative controls, physicians are likely to increase time spent with patients, limit the number of patients they see, and not be concerned about throughput. Physicians paid by capitation are motivated to include as many patients as possible on their patient panel, negotiate a dollar amount per patient that is as high as possible, and perhaps reduce the number of hours they are available to provide care as long as they do not lose patients. For physicians paid on a fee-for-service basis, doing more is better, especially among those performing procedures for which payment is high relative to the amount of labor required. For instance, providing a complex visit vs a simple visit, labeling a wound complex vs simple, or spending more time with a patient under anesthesia all result in increased reimbursement. Thus, physicians have an incentive to provide a longer or more complex service.[1]

Paying physicians by a combination of methods (eg, capitation and fee for service) could, in theory, alter some of the results in the aforementioned examples.[2] Ultimately, however, what a physician does or does not do depends on the Hippocratic Oath, ethics, and morals. Payment mechanisms rarely result in egregious activities that might be considered malpractice, unethical, immoral, or even criminal.

Each mechanism entails risks. A salaried approach may produce too much care for an individual patient and too little for a population. In attempts to increase physician productivity, systems that employ physicians control appointment books, visit length, or the number of hours that a practice needs to be open. When a physician is paid by capitation, underuse can be a problem, so payers or organizations may limit the number of patients that physicians have on their patient panel, arguing that too many patients will result in lower quality.[3]

Under fee-for-service arrangements, the risk is overuse. Efforts to control overuse can take the form of monitoring the number of services a physician provides in a year and paying physicians less per unit of activity to curtail services.

Given these risks, policy makers have become frustrated with these payment mechanisms. This frustration is part of the reason that the US Congress cannot agree on how much to pay physicians under Medicare. Its decision will, of course, affect the amount of money physicians earn. But, in addition, it could alter what physicians do (eg, increase volume of services that are lucrative, divide services into smaller billable packages, or even refuse to take Medicare patients). For those reasons, policy makers have argued that payment mechanisms, such as fee for service, should be supplemented with transparency and pay for performance. Transparency takes the form of publishing the results of physician procedures, in terms of either cost or quality, based on the assumption that patients will choose higher-quality and lower-cost physicians. Pay for performance adds the notion that the probability of achieving certain cost and quality goals is increased by linking lower cost and higher quality to payment.

There has been enough experience to date with pay for performance and transparency to argue convincingly that neither of these additional mechanisms for compensating physicians will achieve the goal of most patients to receive high-quality, humane, and affordable care unless the mechanisms are substantially improved.[4–7] These mechanisms are not silver bullets; they can enhance performance only modestly. They are not capable of improving performance to the level expected of other products such as automobiles. In the vernacular of quality management, these mechanisms cannot, in isolation, achieve "Six Sigma" results.

In addition, these mechanisms may have unintended consequences. For instance, if winning a specific event will bring an elite athlete world recognition, that athlete will design training to win that event. But training for that event may make it more difficult to win a different event. For example, the athlete may need muscle mass for the current challenge but will need flexibility for future competitions. The analogy is apt for pay for performance. If only a few measures are used in pay-for-performance arrangements, clinicians will design particular aspects of their practice to ensure those measures are achieved, even if it means reducing quality of care in other practice areas. Thus, unless the measures used for pay for performance or transparency are comprehensive, these mechanisms can result in unintended and undesirable consequences.

Addressing quality and value in health care delivery would involve ensuring that no matter how physicians are paid, systems designed to achieve value are in place. For example, at the very minimum, physicians in primary care practices should know how many patients they have, who the patients are, and whether the physicians are responsible for both delivering and coordinating all care given to that patient. Physicians should know how much they spend per patient per year and the trend of those expenditures. They should know how many patients in their practice have died and what proportion of deaths is due to medical care that could have been better. Physicians need a system that informs them before they see a patient what unfinished business remains from previous visits, what referrals have not been answered, what laboratory test results have not been examined, and what prescriptions have not been filled. Other functions could be added, with the goal of setting up a health care system that manages the health of a patient population on a real-time basis.

Examples such as these offer insights for designing systems of care and for considering the way physicians are paid. Pay for performance, transparency, and other innovative ways of compensating physicians will work only if, at the same time, the system for providing care is changed to one that has clear objectives and provides specific tools to help physicians achieve those objectives. Otherwise, the new approaches will only increase frustration. At the least, the elements described herein should be considered in policy reform that affects the way physicians are reimbursed for providing care in the developed world.

## References

1. American Medical Association. *Current Procedural Terminology.* Standard ed. Chicago, IL: American Medical Association; 2007.

2. Newhouse JP. *Pricing the Priceless: A Health Care Conundrum.* Cambridge, MA: MIT Press; 2002.

3. Meyer H. Report from the field: Group Health's move to the medical home: for doctors, it's often a hard journey. *Health Aff (Millwood).* 2010;29(5):844-851.

4. Campbell SM, Reeves D, Kontopantelis E, Sibbald B, Roland M. Effects of pay for performance on the quality of primary care in England. *N Engl J Med.* 2009;361(4):368-378.

5. Tu JV, Donovan LR, Lee DS, et al. Effectiveness of public report cards for improving the quality of cardiac care: the EFFECT study: a randomized trial. *JAMA.* 2009;302(21):2330-2337.

6. Hibbard JH, Stockard J, Tusler M. Hospital performance reports: impact on quality, market share, and reputation. *Health Aff (Millwood).* 2005;24(4):1150-1160.

7. Rosenthal MB, Frank RG, Li Z, Epstein AM. Early experience with pay-for-performance: from concept to practice. *JAMA.* 2005;294(14):1788-1793.

# What If Physicians Actually Had to Control Medical Costs?

*Robert H. Brook, MD, ScD*

JAMA, *October 6, 2010—Vol. 304, No. 13, pp. 1489–1490*

What if, at the beginning of a year, a physician were to face the following situation? A physician has been told that enough money is available to treat 100 patients who have either condition A or condition B and treating each patient costs US $1000. Based on epidemiological data, the physician is expected to have 100 patients with condition A and 100 patients with condition B during the calendar year. The health benefit of treating patients with condition A is 4 times as great as the health benefit of treating patients with condition B. There is only $100 000 available, which is only enough money to treat half of the 200 patients.

The first patient the physician observes on the first day of the year has condition B. What does the physician do? Treat the patient, knowing that by the end of the year, she will not be able to offer therapy to at least 1 patient with condition A who seeks care? Do not treat the patient and do not mention that treatment is available? Do not treat the patient, but tell him that he should seek treatment with a different clinician or seek care outside the country? What if the physician got tired of the balancing act and moved to another country or quit working as a physician? Will the above situation actually ever occur? What might physicians do to prevent it?

Policy makers discuss controlling medical costs, and academics publish articles analyzing cost-control approaches. But physicians seem oblivious to the possibility that, sooner or later, care will need to be explicitly rationed. Physicians who actually order the health-related diagnostics or treatment for which taxpayers pay must decide how they will cope with explicit rationing. Will there be a physician plan or health professional plan to deal with the eventuality of explicit rationing? Should planning begin now instead of waiting until the decision is imminent?

Policy makers in virtually every developed country are concerned about the proportion of gross domestic product spent on health care. One response has been to commission studies to change how care is paid for. For example, in the United States, efforts are under way to bundle payment for inpatient and outpatient chronic care.[1] The development of accountable care organizations, medical homes, disease management, and other activities is designed to moderate the growth rate in the proportion of gross domestic product spent on health care and to reduce the amount that federal and state governments spend on health care, so they can avoid raising taxes. Analyses of these options tend to conclude that although they may make some small difference,[2] the relentless growth rate in health care spending will continue, spurred by new medical and biotechnology developments and the aging of the population, among other factors.

What do physicians think about the failure of current cost control strategies and what alternatives can they offer? Currently, very little is known on a population basis about how physicians approach decisions that involve rationing. For example, in a county hospital with limited appointment slots available for patients referred to neurologists, how does the neurologist decide which patients to see? Is the decision based on the length of the note referring the patient, the specificity of the request, the nature of the clinical problem, the personal relationship between the referring physician and the specialist, or other factors?

In an article on how physicians ration health care, Mechanic[3] suggested that physicians do so implicitly because it is just too difficult to do it explicitly. He also suggested that democracy may not be able to support an explicit rationing system.[3] A review of qualitative studies examined how physicians implicitly ration care in individual settings.[4] The studies are not generalizable, but they establish that when confronting time or supply constraints, physicians are making decisions about how to use their time or deciding which patient should receive which test.[4]

The rule regarding how many hours house officers are allowed to be in the hospital was recently changed.[5] How does a resident, required to limit time spent in the hospital to 80 hours in a week, decide with which of the many patients needing care he or she will spend the last hour of the 80-hour week?

Policy makers have attempted to provide some help. Organizations in England, such as the National Institute for Health and Clinical Excellence, have tried to take the decision from the physician and put it squarely on society by implementing a public process to decide what new technologies, devices, or drugs should be part of the benefit package of the National Health Service (NHS).[6] To plan for what was seen as an inevitable reduction in the NHS budget, a series of exercises were conducted to examine the effects of reducing the NHS budget by 10%, or by 20%, or keeping it flat, instead of increasing it at the rate of inflation.[7] The Oregon Medicaid plan went through a similar public process, trying to decide what set of procedures and diagnoses should be covered, given a limited amount of money.[8] Israel and other countries also have formal mechanisms to decide what new medical technology will become part of the benefit package.

In the United States, some explicit programs are in place to help control costs. For example, in pharmacy benefit plans generic drugs are offered at lower co-payments than brand name drugs. Many benefit programs cover only generic equivalents of brand-name drugs. On the other hand, there is an implicit, perhaps irrational, mostly unknown process by which physicians, faced with the everyday pressures of their practices and policy decrees, try to determine how much time to spend with a complex patient, whether there is an appointment slot to schedule a follow-up visit sooner rather than later, who gets which therapy vs another, and how constraints in hospital or nursing home beds or specialty availability can be addressed. These microdecisions play out every day. However, this implicit behavior needs to be integrated with explicit policies. Put more starkly, an explicit plan for rationing needs to be developed. But who will do it, and how?

Every new initiative faces the initial decision of whether that initiative can be pursued free of cost or whether investment is needed to make it happen. It is unlikely that physicians will donate all the time and resources needed to develop a plan for morphing implicit rationing into a more explicit process that is done better. It is also highly unlikely that the US government will pay to develop such a plan. Individual donors are not likely to provide funding because most donors want to increase services and help the needy rather than to understand how rationing medical care can be used to control costs. Thus, it will probably fall upon foundations, brave ones at that, to work with health professionals to begin developing a plan to make rationing of health care explicit and fact based. Physicians need to lead the development of such a plan, and patients and the public must be involved. Basically the plan must provide guidance about what to do in an environment where everything cannot be done for everyone all the time.

Physicians must become a constructive voice in deciding how health care costs can more appropriately reflect society's values and needs. Planning for that eventuality should begin now, but cannot be led by a single specialty organization, cannot aggravate the town/gown split in medicine, cannot conclude by protecting the salaries of physicians relative to the salaries of other health care professionals, and cannot be performed in a way that violates the Hippocratic oath. However, it must be done. At the very least, a set of detailed options needs to be developed to contain costs, and physicians should lead the debate about how such options might be implemented.

There is no group more trusted in society than physicians. If anyone can lead development of such a plan, it should be physicians. US physicians are fortunate to live in a wealthy country that respects democratic processes; therefore, developing cost-control options should be easier than in many other places in the world. Hopefully, by the time health care reform is implemented in 2014, there will be a set of physician plans and options, fully debated, that examine not only how reasonable health care coverage can be provided to everyone, but also how it can be done in a way that is affordable.

## References

1. Health Care and Education Affordability Reconciliation Act of 2010, HR 4872 (2010).

2. Eibner C, Hussey PS, Ridgely MS, McGlynn EA. *Controlling Health Care Spending in Massachusetts: An Analysis of Options.* TR-733-COMMASS. Santa Monica, CA: The RAND Corp; 2009.

3. Mechanic D. Dilemmas in rationing health care services: the case for implicit rationing. *BMJ.* 1995;310(6995):1655-1659.

4. Strech D, Synofzik M, Marckmann G. How physicians allocate scarce resources at the bedside: a systematic review of qualitative studies. *J Med Philos.* 2008;33(1):80-99.

5. *Common Program Requirements: Resident Duty Hours in the Learning and Working Environment.* Chicago, IL: Accreditation Council for Graduate Medical Education; 2007.

6. National Institute for Health and Clinical Excellence. *The Guidelines Manual.* London, England: National Institute for Health and Clinical Excellence; 2009.

7. Harvey S, Liddell A, McMahon L. *Windmill 2009: NHS Response to the Financial Storm.* London, England: King's Fund; 2009.

8. Hadorn DC. The Oregon priority-setting exercise: quality of life and public policy. *Hastings Cent Rep.* 1991;21(3):11-16.

# The End of the Quality Improvement Movement: Long Live Improving Value

*Robert H. Brook, MD, ScD*
*JAMA, October 27, 2010—Vol. 304, No. 16, pp. 1831–1832*

The modern academic quality improvement movement began more than 40 years ago with a series of articles that highlighted substantial deficiencies in the way care was provided.[1] In response, multiple efforts to improve quality were launched. Medical processes that affected patients' health were identified. Methods of measuring how well the processes were performed in day-to-day practice were developed, and many suggestions were made regarding how the processes could be performed better and care improved.

Everyone got into the act. The US government established organizations to review quality of care on an area wide or geographic basis.[2] Hospital accreditation organizations changed their focus from improving the structure of facilities (eg, bricks and mortar, licensure) to what was done to patients, and eventually, to what happened to patients.[3] Organizations were developed to accredit and examine quality of care in the outpatient arena.[4] Hospitals developed quality assurance departments. Organizations such as the Institute for Healthcare Improvement blossomed into leaders in the field of quality improvement, helping institutions provide a better product.[5] Businesses and corporations formed groups to focus the attention of the health care profession on producing a higher-quality product.[6]

More than 40 years later it is unclear what the quality movement has accomplished. Very little is known about how many dollars are invested to improve quality of care nationally or who makes that investment, and there is insufficient evidence about whether or how the quality of care has actually improved. However, what is known is that there is a long way to go.[7] There is no yearly clinically detailed comprehensive report on the epidemiology of quality. Quality can be defined with more reliability and validity, but there is little information about which mechanisms for improving quality work better than others.

More than a decade ago, as the quality improvement movement seemed to stall, many, including the Institute of Medicine, questioned whether the words or concept "quality of health care" had caught the attention of the US public and whether sufficient resources were being invested in the quality movement to actually improve care.

As a result, there was a major effort to relabel and morph the quality improvement movement into the patient safety movement.[8]

The difference between quality and safety is not clear. If a surgeon removes the wrong limb, is that a quality problem or a safety problem? Are errors of commission (ie, placing a feeding tube in the lungs as opposed to the stomach) and errors of omission (ie, failing to give a surgical patient anticoagulation) problems of quality or safety? In any event, refocusing quality to safety seemed to have reenergized the quality improvement movement for a period.

However, the change did not produce the sustained momentum desired by leaders. So the quality improvement movement began to change again. The focus shifted from improving the outcome of care (ie, health of patients) to establishing a business case for quality. The argument was that in most industries improving the quality of the product saved money (fewer recalls, better and less expensive products), so investing in quality of health care should also save money. Organizations and researchers trying to obtain grant funding were asked to demonstrate the business case for quality. Although there are some examples in the literature to support the concept that better quality of care is less expensive, few studies have produced information that could be generalized across time and institutional settings. Indeed, it is the rare article that actually includes measurement of cost or expenditures in a study that attempts to improve quality.[9] Of course, many chief executive officers in organizations from insurance companies to nursing homes invest in and evaluate projects designed both to improve quality and reduce cost. However, the information derived from such activities is not generally in the public domain.

So more than 40 years after the birth of the quality improvement movement, there is still not much known about what has been accomplished. There is little information about whether quality is better in one state or country than another; what the relationship is between the amount a country spends on health care and the quality of care provided in its health care system; whether a business case for quality actually exists in an individual institution or physician's office; and whether the amount of money spent on improving quality is too little or too much.

In addition, there is little debate about how to allocate health care dollars between developing new technologies or improving the quality of care of existing systems. For example, a company develops a new drug that for $30 000 provides one person one good year of life. Such a drug would meet the criteria set by the National Institute for Clinical Excellence (NICE) and would be included in the formulary in the UK's National Health Service (NHS).[10] Would individuals in the NHS have been better off if the funding needed to provide this drug were spent on improving the quality of care given to diabetic children—care that, in turn, could prevent or delay complications? For that matter, there are no publicly available data to answer the question of whether spending $30 000 on quality improvement activities could produce 0, 1, or 100 additional good years of life.

In considering the next 50 years of quality assurance activities, perhaps academics and industry leaders should embrace the business case for quality and focus on the nexus of quality and cost. What is needed is a health care system at the intersection of higher quality and lower cost. In order to get there, the orientation of the entire academic quality field from research to implementation needs to be changed to include cost as well as quality and to understand how to obtain the greatest return for investment.

Instead of trying to fill gaps in knowledge about the epidemiology of quality, the focus should be on developing an epidemiology of value, which contains both measurement of cost and quality, and is applicable to both the developed and developing world. The results of this work would help to distinguish between a level of quality that is a good value and the best available quality that may produce small improvements in health at enormous cost.

Developing such a plan will require much more than current international data comparing life expectancy to total expenditures on health care because much of life expectancy is not under the control of the health care system. For instance, the following types of questions need to be answered. If an individual has a myocardial infarction in London, New York, Los Angeles, or Athens, what is the quality of care he or she will receive, what is the likelihood he or she will survive, and what is the cost in each city for producing that level of quality and that health outcome? Perhaps this exercise would help leaders of hospitals and health systems to make a business case for investing in improving quality.

Facilitating such an agenda will require changing the names of organizations. Organizations with names such as the International Society for Quality in Health Care might change to the International Society for Value in Health Care. Perhaps quality researchers and other individuals who lead quality improvement activities should no longer meet just with their own community, which is mostly concerned with health, but also with managers, economists, and financial experts.

It may be possible to answer questions about what has happened to quality of care in the world in the last 40 years, and at the same time, answer the more difficult question of what investments in quality improvement are worthwhile. Establishing the business case for quality would be a win-win proposition for everyone. Maybe it will lead to more time and money being spent on improving the current system rather than paying for some new products and technologies that are costly and produce only marginal improvements in health.

## References

1. Brook RH, Stevenson RL Jr. Effectiveness of patient care in an emergency room. *N Engl J Med.* 1970;283(17):904-907.

2. Sanazaro PJ, Goldstein RL, Roberts JS, Maglott DB, McAllister JW. Research and development in quality assurance. The experimental medical care review organization program. *N Engl J Med.* 1972;287(22):1125-1131.

3. Roberts JS, Coale JG, Redman RR. A history of the Joint Commission on Accreditation of Hospitals. *JAMA.* 1987;258(7):936-940.

4. Pawlson LG, O'Kane ME. Professionalism, regulation, and the market: impact on accountability for quality of care. *Health Aff (Millwood).* 2002;21(3):200-207.

5. Kenney C. *The Best Practice: How the New Quality Movement Is Transforming Medicine.* New York, NY: Public Affairs; 2008.

6. Galvin RS, Delbanco S, Milstein A, Belden G. Has the leapfrog group had an impact on the health care market? *Health Aff (Millwood).* 2005;24(1):228-233.

7. McGlynn EA, Asch SM, Adams J, et al. The quality of health care delivered to adults in the United States. *N Engl J Med.* 2003;348(26):2635-2645.

8. Kohn LT, Corrigan J, Donaldson MS. *To Err Is Human: Building a Safer Health System.* Washington, DC: National Academies Press; 2000.

9. Ovretveit J. *Does Improving Quality Save Money? A Review of Evidence of Which Improvements to Quality Reduce Costs to Health Service Providers.* London, UK: The Health Foundation; 2009.

10. Rawlins MD, Culyer AJ. National Institute for Clinical Excellence and its value judgments. *BMJ.* 2004;329(7459):224-227.

# A Physician = Emotion + Passion + Science

*Robert H. Brook, MD, ScD*
*JAMA, December 8, 2010—Vol. 304, No. 22, pp. 2528–2529*

Pick up *JAMA* or *The Annals of Internal Medicine*, and what do you notice? The cover of *JAMA* is selected with meticulous detail and tells a story relevant to the world, to medicine, and to the right brain. Both journals devote space to something more personal than a scientific article: in the case of *JAMA*, "A Piece of My Mind" and in the case of the *Annals of Internal Medicine*, "On Being a Doctor." There is even a place for poetry written by physicians. It is not clear how many physicians actually read their copy of *JAMA* or the *Annals of Internal Medicine* when they receive it, but it would be interesting to know how many of them read the sections that appeal to emotion, passion, and the right brain. In "A Piece of My Mind" or "On Being a Doctor," the reader confronts a personal story written in the first person with undisguised emotions—passionate and compelling. Often the stories connect the reader with parts of medicine that have confronted every physician: death, dying, the nontypical patient, one's own frailty, or one's own health.

These personal stories comprise only a minor element in these scholarly journals. But most journals have no such element. No matter how diligently the science contained in the journals has been reviewed, no matter how aggressive the editors have been in identifying topics and work relevant to the practice of medicine, the scientific articles are written in a manner that, in many instances, adopts a bland, somnolent tone. The language has no passion, conveys no emotion. The words stimulate no visual image. Physicians have been taught to present their science in what is called a "flat manner": let the facts speak for themselves. Get rid of adverbs and adjectives, pictures, first person, and just let the science sing.

However, science rarely sings. What if science were presented in the same passionate, emotional style as in those accounts of personal experiences that moved the physician who wrote them? Instead of requiring a science article to have the standard introductory, methods, results, and discussion sections with a certain number of words and a certain number of tables, science articles should perhaps include cartoons, pictures, or emotional images that contain meaning and require the use of both the right and left brain. Perhaps permitting the personal would not degrade the scientific process but rather increase the likelihood that the information contained in the journals would actually be read, absorbed, and used.[1]

Not very long ago, most of the practice of medicine was really about the information contained in the "A Piece of My Mind" or "On Being a Doctor" sections of the journals. There was very little science or technology that made a lot of a difference. Each patient was an individual with a family and a community. Each physician was an individual with a small amount of technology at his or her disposal. Every patient required a different art of care, whether it was the way the patient was touched by the physician or the manner in which experiences were shared or questions were asked. Without available or sufficient health insurance, physicians and patients had to work together to produce treatment plans that were consistent with the patients' culture and socioeconomic status and that reflected the patients' values about the kind of care they wanted and did not want.

That relationship between the physician and the patient changed. Although there was always a desire to remain healthy, as the science and technology of medicine improved, both physicians and patients wanted to take advantage of those potential health benefits. As technology continues to improve, contact with patients becomes more standardized. Procedures and tests are now easier to perform and do not require an artist to accomplish them; rather, they require someone who follows guidelines and operational manuals to make sure that the process of medicine is standardized so that maximum health benefits can be obtained. Thus, it is not unexpected that the communication of scientific advances in medicine would also become standardized, emotionless, and dispassionate.

However, the world of communication has changed. Today, the Internet, Facebook, LinkedIn, and all sorts of connected devices allow humans to immediately share photographs, emotions, thoughts, and passions. It is difficult to imagine a young physician growing up in this communication environment, trying to focus his or her brain on science studies that seem to be written in a language as foreign as medieval English would be to modern inhabitants of the British Isles.

Can anything be done about this? Can information be conveyed with both scientific accuracy and with readability for the next generation of physicians? It would be interesting to experiment with a process that puts passion, emotion, and science together in a new way, producing peer-reviewed, objective information that is consistent with the experiences of the new generation of physicians and clinicians now being trained. It would be nice if the arrival of *JAMA* or the *Annals of Internal Medicine* at the door prompted curiosity and anticipation rather than, perhaps, a sense of duty.

Perhaps some baby steps can be taken. The last paragraph of a scientific article could contain a paragraph in the first-person that reflected feelings. For example, after publishing the results from the RAND Health Insurance Experiment, I was sad.[2] My coauthors and I demonstrated that providing care free to patients did not improve their health any more than did the care for which they paid a portion. Why was the medical care system so sloppy and chaotic that more care did not lead to better health? I was angry that I would spend part of my life defending co-payments because the American public could not be offered a system in which care was free at the point of service and actually produced better health.

If I had written an article for the "A Piece of My Mind" section, it would have been about watching my mother die from old age slowly at home. After sharing that each visit ended with tears, I would like to have asked a question about the science of dying. Can social isolation be reduced at the end of life? Can better systems of dying be put in place? Is everyone going to die in isolation? Is there a science of feeling at the end of life?

Medicine needs to be scientifically based, but physicians need to be engaged through their passions and emotions. The process of medical education can be redesigned to pay attention to all these desirable qualities simultaneously. The type of passionate, emotional, and personal messages conveyed in "A Piece of My Mind" or "On Being a Doctor" need not be a separate department in a journal, kept distinct from discussion of a new advance in the clinical practice of medicine.

## References

1. Shermer MB. This view of science: Stephen Jay Gould as historian of science and scientific historian, popular scientist and scientific popularizer. *Soc Stud Sci*. 2002;32(4):489-524.

2. Brook RH, Ware JE Jr, Rogers WH, et al. Does free care improve adults' health? results from a randomized controlled trial. *N Engl J Med*. 1983;309(23):1426-1434.

# Is Choice of Physician and Hospital an Essential Benefit?

*Robert H. Brook, MD, ScD*
JAMA, *January 12, 2011—Vol. 305, No. 2, pp. 195–196*

In the 1970s, health care was simpler. The fields of transplant surgery, clinical pharmacology, and clinical oncology, among others, were just emerging. The proportion of the gross national product spent on health care was in the low single digits. There were no preferred provider organizations, no publicly available data indicating which surgeon was better than another, no evidence-based medicine movement, or any other kind of information designed to help individuals make treatment choices. In the 1970s, it was reasonable for health insurance to cover the entire gamut of health care, from what currently would be called complementary and alternative medicine to traditional medicine. For those with health insurance, no matter what kind of service a physician and patient agreed to, the service was covered without either evidence that it was effective or prior authorization.

Forty years later, the Patient Protection and Affordable Care Act[1] requires that the federal government define an essential benefit package for those individuals who will obtain insurance through the new health insurance exchanges. The Secretary of the Department of Health and Human Services has asked the Institute of Medicine to assist in this activity.[2]

What is an essential benefit package? One definition is a package that covers anything a physician and patient want, regardless of whether there is clinical evidence to support its use. Patients might be asked to share some portion of the cost of the package benefit, which would help to control use. Cost sharing is effective in reducing the amount of care used. But as the RAND Health Insurance Experiment of the 1970s demonstrated, cost sharing neither changed the quality of care that was delivered, nor did it change whether patients went to physicians for conditions that really required medical care.[3] Stated another way, cost sharing exerted some control on the amount of care used, but it did not change the mix of appropriate or inappropriate care that was used, or improve the quality of care that was provided. Even free care did not affect the mix of care or quality.[3]

So how should an essential benefit be designed in an era when health care is far more expensive, the number of tests and procedures is significantly greater, and evidence-based medicine is the slogan of the day? In addition, consumers have access, at least in theory, to data describing the quality of hospitals, physicians, and health care facilities, complicating discussions regarding what is an essential benefit.

What do individuals want in health care? Obviously, they want to receive the treatment or procedure that can best help to improve their health status. Individuals do not want medical services that are not needed, but they do want those that are. Most individuals probably prefer not to travel very far to obtain needed care. Furthermore, many may ask whether, if given the opportunity, they should seek care from the physician they know or are referred to, or whether they should choose a "better" physician in their local area, or even travel to a health facility such as one of the top-rated hospitals in the country to receive the required procedure, operation, or treatment. Whatever their choice, patients want to be treated humanely—to be respected as individuals and dealt with equitably and compassionately.

This is the complicated context in which health care reform is being implemented and an essential benefit plan is being defined. As the definition process moves forward, answers will be needed for questions that may be uncomfortable to discuss openly, such as whether expensive but marginally effective procedures or medicines should be covered. Another issue is whether an essential benefit package should allow patients to choose where and from whom they receive care with no financial consequences of their decision. Should an essential benefit plan allow this choice only if evidence shows that more expensive physicians and hospitals improve health status and outcomes more than those that are less expensive? What will happen if a patient has reliable information that a particular hospital provides a specific treatment better, or perhaps even far better, than the hospital covered in the patient's essential benefit plan? Will the patient have any recourse? How can patients be empowered and costs be controlled at the same time?

What are the precedents set elsewhere for essential health care benefits? Some countries that provide citizens with basic health care packages do not include choice of either physician or hospital as part of the essential benefit plan. In Israel, for example, a patient has to pay more for the privilege of choosing a specific surgeon.[4]

The following illustration makes these issues more concrete. A middle-aged man has a condition that meets evidence-based criteria for having coronary artery bypass graft surgery. If he undergoes the operation performed by the best surgeon in his local area or in his region of the country, he will be less likely to die. For example, depending on the patient's health, his expected death rate would be 1% not 2%.[5] The patient's health plan, in theory, allows him to make such choices, but the choice is associated with additional cost. After having had a quantitative decision-analytical conversation with his trusted, evidence-based practicing physician in his medical home or accountable health care organization about the adverse effects and the benefits of the procedure, and after reading information on a trustworthy publicly available Web site, the patient decides that he wants to undergo the operation performed by the better surgeon, as defined by available data. However, his health plan requires him to pay an additional $20 000 to have that surgeon do the procedure in the selected hospital, relative to his cost at the hospital in his essential benefit plan. Would this financial burden change the decision?

The Affordable Care Act will add a large number of US citizens to the Medicaid system. When the total number of Medicaid beneficiaries is added to the number of individuals whose health care will be provided by the new insurance exchanges, it becomes clear that what the government chooses to do in defining an essential benefit package will significantly shape both the public and private medical market. It is not sufficient to say that the package will only cover care that evidence shows will benefit the patient. If the available evidence compares one physician or hospital with another, will the same evidence-based principles be applied in defining an essential benefit package? Sports enthusiasts know that whenever a professional athlete is injured, the athlete will seek care for the injury from the best clinician at the best clinic. There is no question about who should perform the needed procedure. As health care reform is implemented, average US citizens will be asking: Is the essential benefit package good enough to protect them and their family and help them live a healthy life? In other words, can the patient and family be certain that they can afford the best hospital or physician if the choice might make a meaningful difference in health?

Individuals cannot predict what procedures they will need, or whether receiving care from a better physician or hospital is potentially life-saving. But if an empowered individual takes the time to access reliable Web sites providing information about the quality of needed care, should acting on such information be discouraged by financial consequences that are part of an essential benefit plan? If the answer is yes, then the movement toward reporting results of surgeons and hospitals will probably lead to a society in which the wealthy receive care from the better hospitals and physicians, and they know it.

# References

1. Eibner C, Hussey PS, Girosi F. The effects of the Affordable Care Act on workers' health insurance coverage. *N Engl J Med*. 2010;363(15):1393-1395.

2. US National Academies Press. Project: defining and revising an essential health benefits package for qualified health plans 2010. http://www8.nationalacademies.org/cp/projectview.aspx?key=IOM-HCS-10-04. Accessed November 29, 2010.

3. Newhouse JP, Rand Corporation Insurance Experiment Group. *Free for All?* Cambridge, MA: Harvard University Press; 1993.

4. European Observatory on Health Care Systems. *Health Care Systems in Transition*. Copenhagen, Denmark: European Observatory on Health Care Systems; 2009.

5. State of California Office of Statewide Health Planning and Development. *Report on Coronary Artery Bypass Graft Surgery 2005-2006 Hospital and Surgeon Data*. Sacramento, CA: Office of Statewide Health Planning and Development; 2009.

# Health Services Research and Clinical Practice

*Robert H. Brook, MD, ScD*
*JAMA, April 20, 2011—Vol. 305, No. 15, pp. 1589–1590*

Health services research is "a multidisciplinary field of scientific investigation that studies how social factors, financing systems, organizational structures and processes, health technologies, and personal behaviors affect access to healthcare, the quality and cost of health care, and ultimately our health and well-being."[1] During the last 50 years, health service researchers have developed tools and techniques that have profoundly affected the way medicine is practiced. The field developed measures of health and quality and ways to incorporate risk adjustment as a function of the characteristics that patients bring to a clinical encounter. These techniques have made it possible to increase measures of health as outcomes in clinical trials and to pay physicians based on their performance. Health services research has built an empirical foundation for empowering patients by providing information that compares quality of care or health outcomes across hospitals or physicians.

What health services research has not done is revolutionize the way medicine is practiced to increase its value and to moderate costs. The United States spends more than 17% of its gross national product on health care[2]; understandably, individuals and families are concerned that health care in the future will be unaffordable. Policy makers are struggling to bend the cost curve by fundamentally altering how physicians and hospitals deliver care. These efforts assume the existence of a comprehensive science-based framework at the patient-physician level that can be used to change the way medicine is practiced. However, such a framework does not exist. The health services research community and practitioners in academic medical centers have tried to address the issue of value in health care, but their efforts have been focused primarily at the level of a single research grant. An integrated effort is needed that crosses specialties, diseases, and conditions, enabling physicians to help bring about the necessary changes.

The purpose of this Commentary is to urge development of an active coalition between leaders in clinical practice and health services researchers to address 5 issues essential for radically changing the practice of medicine: reliability, appropriateness, frequency, labor, and transparency.

## Reliability

Many clinical processes and their health outcomes are not reliable.[3,4] For example, if 2 physicians listen to a patient's heart, do they hear the same thing? If they read the results of a coronary angiography, are their readings consistent?[5] Numerous isolated studies have focused on reliability, but there is no integrated science of reliability or a process for incorporating findings from individual studies into clinical practice. A method is needed to ensure that the information used to inform clinical decision making is reliably collected and interpreted. The need is particularly acute because the field of diagnostics will expand substantially in the next 5 years, and the number of diagnostic tests will increase significantly. Wider use of electronic medical records also increases the importance of improving reliability.

## Appropriateness

Assuming physicians have reliable information, how can this information be used to make decisions about appropriateness? Studies documenting inappropriate care are published frequently. For instance, a recent report suggested that among patients who received an implantable cardioverter-defibrillator, approximately 1 in 5 did not meet evidence-based criteria supporting use of these devices.[6] But these data are based on isolated studies. Clinical practice has not changed to address concerns about appropriateness across multiple procedures and tests.

## Frequency

There is virtually no information about how often any medical test or treatment should be performed. For example, how frequently should blood pressure be monitored or mammograms performed, or how much radiation is necessary to control a tumor? The question of frequency cuts across every branch of medicine, but there is virtually no science of frequency to draw on for answers. Reducing the frequency of performing some medical procedures could eliminate shortages of equipment and professionals. If information were more reliable, health outcomes might be the same even though the frequency of follow-up tests and procedures was reduced.

## Labor

Labor represents another major issue for the medical profession. What kind of care can safely be delivered by nonphysicians? In every aspect of medicine there are examples of procedures that do not require a physician. For example, must the primary care physician be the motivational coach who urges patients to exercise and lose weight? Can a computer that recognizes patterns partially replace specialists? A science that specifies the training necessary for certain clinical activities is needed.

## Transparency

Clinical leaders and health services researchers need to know how far transparency and patient empowerment will evolve and how care will be affected by public dissemination of data about the performance of individual physicians and hospitals. The consumer movement in medicine is now in its infancy and focused primarily on a few aspects of quality of care, but by 2020, patient information, possibly including prices, will determine the framework within which patients and physicians interact.

## Moving Forward

Substantial courage will be needed to pursue this agenda. The interests supporting the status quo are formidable. Not all individuals support the status quo for business reasons, and most physicians do not want to change the way they interact with patients. But how medicine is practiced must change in a way that fosters close collaboration between the research community and the clinical community so that resistance does not become clinicians' operating mode.

   An example of reluctance to change is the medical profession's reaction to the extensive body of research focused on appropriateness of care—work suggesting that a substantial percentage of care was either inappropriate or equivocal. This work was published in major medical journals around the world.[7,8] But physicians did not embrace the findings and modify the way they practiced medicine. Instead, they reaffirmed their commitment to doing exactly what they had been doing. Ironically, insurance carriers adopted the appropriateness techniques and developed utilization review procedures to control what physicians did by controlling what would be compensated. How different the world would be if a collaborative, empowered group of researchers and medical leaders had worked together before the appropriateness work was published so that the results were instantly adopted, thus increasing reliability.

   It is time for medicine to reinvent itself—for researchers and clinicians to form a strategic partnership and to embrace the goal of exponentially increasing medicine's value. Physicians need to become part of the solution in the US health care system. The system's problems should not be addressed by politicians, who are virtually powerless to effect meaningful change in health care until physicians fix the way care is delivered.

   How physicians provide care for patients has to become more reliable, more appropriate, and more transparent. In addition, high-quality care needs to be delivered by professionals with the appropriate level of training and education so that each professional can practice at the top of his or her knowledge base.

## References

1. Lohr KN, Steinwachs DM. Health services research: an evolving definition of the field. *Health Serv Res.* 2002;37(1):7-9.

2. Keehan S, Sisko A, Truffer C, et al; National Health Expenditure Accounts Projections Team. Health spending projections through 2017: the baby-boom generation is coming to Medicare. *Health Aff (Millwood).* 2008;27(2):w145-w155.

3. Koran LM. The reliability of clinical methods, data and judgments (first of two parts). *N Engl J Med.* 1975;293(13):642-646.

4. Koran LM. The reliability of clinical methods, data and judgments (second of two parts). *N Engl J Med.* 1975;293(14):695-701.

5. Leape LL, Park RE, Bashore TM, Harrison JK, Davidson CJ, Brook RH. Effect of variability in the interpretation of coronary angiograms on the appropriateness of use of coronary revascularization procedures. *Am Heart J.* 2000;139(1 pt 1): 106-113.

6. Al-Khatib SM, Hellkamp A, Curtis J, et al. Non-evidence-based ICD implantations in the United States. *JAMA.* 2011;305(1):43-49.

7. Chassin MR, Kosecoff J, Park RE, et al. Does inappropriate use explain geographic variation in the use of health care services? a study of three procedures. *JAMA.* 1987;258(18):2533-2537.

8. Brook RH, Chassin MR, Fink A, Solomon DH, Kosecoff J, Park RE. A method for the detailed assessment of the appropriateness of medical technologies. *Int J Technol Assess Health Care.* 1986;2(1):53-63.

# Accountable Care Organizations and Community Empowerment

*Benjamin F. Springgate, MD, MPH (Tulane University School of Medicine)*
*Robert H. Brook, MD, ScD (RAND Corporation)*
*JAMA, May 4, 2011—Vol. 305, No. 17, pp. 1800–1801*

Implementation of the Affordable Care Act and health care reform is under way. A central dimension of this process that has captured health sector interest is development and implementation of accountable care organizations (ACOs). ACOs are formal collaborations of health care professionals who agree to assume responsibility for providing a specific and potentially comprehensive set of health care services to a defined population of at least 5000 Medicare recipients. ACOs are considered to have the potential to reconfigure care-delivery systems to align incentives among physicians, other health professionals, hospitals, and payers (primarily the federal government through Medicare and the federal share of Medicaid) with the goal of increasing perceived value of care, improving clinical outcomes, and lowering health care costs (the triple aim).[1] The Centers for Medicare & Medicaid Services has indicated that the secretary of the Department of Health and Human Services will share some portion of savings derived from lower costs of ACO care with ACO clinicians.[2]

Less apparent to the public during this period of historic change are the struggles occurring in US board rooms among hospital groups, specialty physicians, and primary care clinicians—debating quietly but intensely over how to form these ACOs, how to be accountable for care delivery, and how to divide anticipated savings derived from ACOs. However, in most of these settings, important constituencies—middle class and other working patients whose health and welfare are at stake—are not included in the discussions.

This suggests a number of provocative speculations. Would the discussions be any different if this community of patients participated as equal principals in forming ACOs alongside their physicians and hospital representatives? In many ways, the ACOs proposed today were anticipated by the models of community-oriented primary care debated nearly 3 decades ago except that community-oriented primary care more explicitly expected "involvement of the community in the promotion of its health."[3] Group Health Cooperative, a Puget Sound health care system, well known for high quality of care, has for nearly as long ensured community involvement and leadership through its elected patient board and patient councils.[4]

If presented with the option, would communities of patients require specific benefits, roles, and responsibilities in exchange for participating in an ACO? Would the behaviors of community members resemble those of blocs of shareholders in a corporation, partners in a group venture, or patient-board members of neighborhood health centers? Would this kind of patient relationship with the formal care delivery system potentially change the social contract of health care delivery and increase the likelihood of achieving the triple aim, ie, improving the health of the population, enhancing the patient experience of care, and reducing or controlling the per capita cost of health care[1] or some piece of it? Would communities of patient shareholders perceive each of these aims as equally relevant or valuable? Would they perceive the aims in the same way or differently from how they are perceived by provider groups? Might engaged and empowered communities be more motivated to work with clinicians to receive needed health care services or to engage in health-promoting behaviors if granted an equitable voice in discussions about how the health care system to which they subscribe is configured and implemented?

Would it make a difference if that opportunity came now, before the ACOs have been fully developed, as opposed to bringing in these communities as partners after the ACO was already functioning? Would this opportunity to participate in decision making—to argue, to vote, to express opinion freely about an individual's own health care system in a forum with real power—have an effect on health and potentially represent a step toward more effective and more patient-centered care? The freedom of individuals to participate in decisions that have significant influence on their lives has been proposed as an important way to improve health and economic functioning.[5]

Similarly, patients are believed to benefit from playing active roles in health care choices and decision making. Patient-centered medical homes have been widely promoted in recent years as a means to achieve improved health outcomes and enhance patient participation in care.[6] Yet, programs that formally recognize patient-centered medical homes may not require any input from patients in the recognition process.[7] Analogous assessment programs are currently under consideration for the evaluation of ACOs.[8] Might an ACO be more cost-effective if a majority of the community of patient-shareholders routinely reviewed independent measurements of quality of care and expenditure decisions and provided guidance to the ACO's management?

As an alternative, some communities of patients may be more motivated to contribute to improved health care outcomes and cost savings by the opportunity to receive a monetary return on their investment of active participation in an ACO. Such incentives appear to work well for physicians and hospital groups—why not for patients? A part of shared savings returned to an ACO might be divided with participating groups of patients. Perhaps this portion of the shared savings could even be construed as a tax refund for the patient-shareholders. Few would argue against aligning financial interests to improve outcomes while also lowering the effective tax rate.

It is possible that financial return on community-shareholder participation would indirectly promote choices of healthful activities such as community decisions to invest in fresh produce markets or to purchase group memberships in exercise programs. Perhaps specific groups of Medicare patients would reinvest the ACO savings in group shareholder benefits such as lower medication co-pays, or a patient-accessible community center with a gymnasium where none currently exists.

Are such visions of community engagement in health care unrealistic or already emerging in ways that even a few months ago could not have been imagined? For instance, opportunities for communities of patients to make their voices heard have increased dramatically, aided in part by social media and participatory technologies such as Facebook, Twitter, short-message service (SMS) text, and e-mail. Can communities of patient-shareholders be recruited to join an ACO and can their involvement in ACOs effectively be operationalized? Would physicians and hospitals even permit such a dramatic step toward more patient-centered care?

The high and accelerating increases in the cost of health care and the limited roles of patients in decision making central to health and health care delivery are too real to ignore. Decision making by distal proxies such as elected legislators may no longer be enough to address the United States' mounting problems with health care, outcomes, and costs.

## References

1. Berwick DM, Nolan TW, Whittington J. The triple aim: care, health, and cost. *Health Aff (Millwood)*. 2008;27(3):759-769.

2. Centers for Medicare & Medicaid Services. Medicare accountable care organizations: shared savings program—new Section 1899 of Title XVIII, preliminary questions and answers. https://www.cms.gov/OfficeofLegislation/Downloads/AccountableCareOrganization.pdf. Accessed February 16, 2011.

3. Connor E, Mullan F. *Community Oriented Primary Care: New Directions for Health Services Delivery*. Washington, DC: National Academy Press; 1983.

4. Emanuel EJ, Emanuel LL. Preserving community in health care. *J Health Polit Policy Law*. 1997;22(1):147-184.

5. Sen A. *Development as Freedom*. New York, NY: Alfred A Knopf; 1999.

6. American Academy of Family Physicians; American Academy of Pediatrics; American College of Physicians; American Osteopathic Association. Joint principles of the patient-centered medical home: February 2007. http://www.aafp.org/online /etc/medialib/aafp_org/documents/policy/fed/jointprinciplespcmh0207.Par.0001.File.dat/022107medicalhome.pdf. Accessed February 16, 2011.

7. National Committee for Quality Assurance. Patient-centered medical home. http://www.ncqa.org/tabid/74/Default.aspx. Accessed February 16, 2011.

8. National Committee for Quality Assurance. Accountable care organizations (ACO): draft 2011 criteria. http://www.ncqa.org/portals/0/publiccomment/ACO/ACO_%20Overview.pdf. Accessed February 16, 2011.

# Facts, Facts, Facts: What Is a Physician to Do?

*Robert H. Brook, MD, ScD*

JAMA, *July 27, 2011—Vol. 306, No. 4, pp. 432–433*

It is a cliché to observe that everyone lives in a global economy. Anyone who travels internationally can see how rapidly the world is becoming similar in terms of shops, goods, and services. Perhaps it is timely to reengage physicians in the discussion of international comparative data about health care and to ask why the United States is so provincial in designing the systems by which care is delivered.

Recently the Organisation for Economic Co-operation and Development (OECD) published Health at a Glance 2009,[1] the annual compilation of health statistics from 30 countries. Even though most of the data are from 2007, these statistics provide revealing snapshots of various aspects of health and health systems, especially when comparing several US statistics to comparable statistics from other countries.

Seventeen comparisons were selected to be representative of the different concepts (health status, nonmedical determinants of health, health work force, health care activities, quality of care, and health expenditures) that are covered in the OECD report. The comparisons (reported as United States; another country) are as follows.

1. Life expectancy in the United States is 78.1 years; in Switzerland, it is 81.9 years.[1(pp15-41)]

2. Years of life lost before age 70 per 100 000 men is 6291; in Italy, it is 3605.[1(pp15-41)]

3. The age-standardized ischemic heart mortality rate per 100 000 males is 145; in France, it is 54.[1(pp15-41)]

4. The percentage of newborns weighing less than 2500 g is 8.3%; in Ireland, it is 5%.[1(pp15-41)]

5. The percentage of children aged 11 to 15 years who are overweight or obese is 29.8%; in Belgium, it is 10.5%.[1(pp43-57)]

6. The number of practicing physicians per 1000 population is 2.4; in Belgium, it is 4.0.[1(pp59-85)]

7. The percentage of US physicians who are non-US trained is 25.9%; in the Netherlands, the percentage of non-Netherlands–trained physicians is 6.3%.[1(pp59-85)]

8. The ratio of the self-employed specialist's average salary to the average salary of a full-time employee is 5.6:1; in Germany, the ratio is 4.1:1. For a self-employed general practitioner, the comparable ratio is 3.7:1; in Canada, it is 3.1:1.[1(pp59-85)]

9. The number of physician consultations per capita is 3.8; in Germany, it is 7.5, and in Japan, it is 13.6.[1(pp87-109)]

10. The number of consultations per physician per year (data are from administrative sources and include visits in physician offices, hospital outpatient clinics, or patient homes) is 1570; in Korea, it is 7251 and in Canada, it is 3335 (fee-for-service visits only).[1(pp87-109)]

11. The number of magnetic resonance imaging (MRI) machines per 1 000 000 of population is 25.9; in Japan, it is 40.1; in Canada, it is 6.7.[1(pp87-109)]

12. The number of MRI examinations per 1000 population is 91.2; in Canada, the number is 31.2.[1(pp87-109)]

13. The hospital discharge rate is 126 per 1000; in France, it is 274.[1(pp87-109)]

14. The coronary revascularization rate is 521 per 100 000; in Switzerland, it is 144 and in Ireland, it is 128.[1(pp87-109)]

15. The number of patients treated for end-stage renal failure is 169 per 100 000 population; in the Netherlands, it is 77.[1(pp87-109)]

16. The age-sex standardized in-hospital death rate for acute myocardial infarction is 5.1%; in Sweden, it is 2.9%.[1(pp111-137)]

17. Health expenditures are 16.0% of gross domestic product; in France, 11% and in Ireland, 7.6%.[1(pp157-173)]

What might physicians do with these or other similar data? Physicians have shown little interest in this kind of documented variation in health care systems within a country, let alone across 30 countries. Perhaps it is time to reduce that indifference. When medical societies debate the number of fellowships or residency positions needed, perhaps they should take heed of the international data. Perhaps MRI purchase decisions in the United States should be informed by some understanding of the role that MRIs play in other countries. How do other countries manage to reduce the number of individuals receiving renal dialysis or undergoing revascularization procedures or to decrease the mortality rate from myocardial infarction? Should anyone in the United States care that a physician in Korea manages 7251 patient visits in 1 year?

Clients of the OECD are the governments of its member countries. The question is whether government ministers of health can use OECD data to produce a better health care system when physicians ignore the data.

Advances in electronic medical records and information sciences will exponentially increase the amount of comparative data that can be produced across countries. Physicians should help to direct the type of data collected and to increase the validity and reliability of these data. At the same time, there needs to be a more open exploration of what data suggest about how the US health care system is performing and how it can be improved.

In this Commentary, the United States is compared with individual countries rather than to the mean of the OECD 30-country sample. This was done because each of the countries with which the United States was compared has a different type of health care system, a different culture, different population characteristics, and different ways of delivering clinical care. Any of these factors could contribute to the differences reflected in the OECD data.

Using these data wisely to improve health and health care requires physician input and leadership. Future international comparisons should include actionable tasks that physicians believe should be pursued to reduce cross-country variations in health outcomes, to eliminate waste, and to increase value and improve health. Perhaps there is a right rate for MRIs per person or patient visits per physician. Perhaps reducing variation in life expectancy per country can be achieved by physicians assuming a leadership role in examining these data and then altering the clinical methods used. Perhaps in the near future, when the attending physician making hospital rounds says that the US population is exposed to 3 times the number of MRIs than the Canadian population, the statement will be followed with a clinical explanation and a call for action. It should be known at a clinical level why these rates differ and which, if any, are more appropriate. This can be done only with physician input.

## Reference

1. Organisation for Economic Co-operation and Development. *Health at a Glance 2009*. Paris, France: Organisation for Economic Co-operation and Development; 2009. doi:10.1787/health_glance-2009-en

# The Role of Physicians in Controlling Medical Care Costs and Reducing Waste

*Robert H. Brook, MD, ScD*
*JAMA, August 10, 2011—Vol. 306, No. 6, pp. 650–651*

The looming US budget crisis figures prominently in daily news. The amount of money spent on medical care is increasing faster than the gross domestic product (GDP), and the federal deficit is increasing. Budget experts believe that the deficit cannot be reduced unless medical spending can be controlled. What role will physicians play in controlling health care cost growth? Are physicians even willing to play a role?

Realistically, physicians face 3 scenarios in controlling health care costs. In the first scenario, physicians do nothing. Cost increases continue unabated and the proportion of GDP spent on health care continues to increase. But sooner or later, with or without the help of physicians, the cost crisis will have to be confronted. In a crisis mode, the solution to the spending problem may not be what physicians, or their patients, want.

In the second scenario, health care is rationed. When the "R" word is mentioned, all rational discussion ceases, but the inexorable production of devices, drugs, and procedures that generates both health benefits and higher costs may eventually force the rationing decision.[1] There are multiple ways of implementing rationing, but most individuals would like to prevent it.

In the third scenario, physicians take the lead in identifying and eliminating waste in US health care. Physicians could define waste by assigning all services to 1 of 4 types of care—inappropriate, equivocal, appropriate, or necessary. With inappropriate care, the potential health benefit to the patient is less than the potential harm caused by the procedure, device, or drug. With equivocal care, potential harm and benefit are about equal. With appropriate care, potential benefit to the patient exceeds potential harm. Necessary care is appropriate, represents the only viable option, and produces a large health benefit.

An economist would define waste differently. Waste to an economist is an expenditure that does not produce commensurate value. Many economists believe that the value of a human life is at least $3 million, if not twice that.[2] Therefore, care that provides 1 good year of quality life and costs less than $50,000 to $100,000 is not wasteful,[2] but care that produces a year of good life and costs more than $150,000 is wasteful. Physicians prefer the medical definition. But it is not known how much clinical waste is in the system.

For example, consider the best performing hospitals or health systems in the United States, defined by some measure of quality or efficiency. Based on either metric, how much waste is there in those hospitals or health systems? To answer this question, a tool is needed to measure clinical waste. A comprehensive tool to measure waste across all clinical services does not exist today, but there are many tools that focus on certain aspects of care. After a more complete tool is developed, patients treated in the best performing hospitals or health systems could be sampled after stratifying them based on the total amount of money they spent on health care anywhere in a given year. After the sample is selected, each patient's medical record could be reviewed and each service received assigned to 1 of the 4 categories (inappropriate, equivocal, appropriate, or necessary).

It would not be very expensive to conduct this review of records for a reasonable sample of patients. The result would be a rough estimate of the potential waste in the system—that is, the proportion of services that were in the inappropriate or equivocal categories. If circumstances demanded, the definition of waste could be expanded to any service that was not in the necessary category.

Once the proportion of care in each category is determined, what portion of health care costs is associated with each category could be determined. In doing this, how eliminating wasteful services affects short-term costs, long-term costs, fixed costs, average costs, and marginal costs could be assessed. In addition, if wasteful services are eliminated, necessary services that the patient did not receive might need to be added (eg, angioplasty is eliminated for a patient with stable angina but additional medical therapy is required). The cost of these additional necessary services would need to be deducted from the previous estimate of savings.

This process would generate an estimate of the proportion of care in top-performing hospitals or health systems that is wasteful and the amount of money that could be saved if clinical methods were improved. If the work is performed correctly, it might even be possible to assign ranges and confidence intervals to the estimates.

Some individuals may be more comfortable sampling care in average hospitals and health care systems. Whatever the sample, if the proportion of care estimated to be wasteful comprises only a small percentage of total costs, then eliminating waste is not a promising policy option for cost containment.

Delivery of health care in the United States is entering troubled waters. There are proposals being considered to roll back government-sponsored health insurance[3] and proposals to limit the benefits individuals have under health insurance.[4] It is unclear whether any of these proposals would have political traction if the US government did not have an enormous budget deficit, driven by uncontrolled Medicaid and Medicare expenditures. The next political window regarding the future of the US health care system is likely to open right after the next presidential election. Before draconian measures are enacted, the waste question needs a scientific answer that physicians agree is valid and reliable.

Physicians should not be taken by surprise. If physicians can help reduce the budget deficit by eliminating waste in the health care system, the profession must agree on what proportion of care is wasteful. Better would be to identify strategies for eliminating waste within a very few years. Such strategies must include teaching all physicians how to recognize and eliminate clinical waste. Board certification examinations and tests in medical school could require physicians to separate waste from necessary care and demonstrate that they use such knowledge in day-to-day practice. Board certified physicians could represent only those physicians who not only provide high-quality care, but do so with minimal amounts of waste. Hospitals viewed as the country's best could be those hospitals that reduce clinical waste to a minimum. Without agreement within the medical profession about the magnitude of clinical waste, physicians cannot hope to have a strong influence in the health care cost debate.

In this Commentary, waste has been defined as the use of clinical services that cannot be classified as necessary or necessary and appropriate, but there are other definitions of waste. For example, a service could be defined as wasteful if it is performed by someone with a high salary, when it could be performed with the same outcome by someone who is paid less. Similarly, it is wasteful for a physician to perform a service that a computer could perform at a lower cost with equivalent outcomes, or for a necessary service to be delivered inefficiently. Such considerations have been excluded not because they are unimportant, but because the first step must be to reach agreement on which clinical services, under what circumstances, currently being provided are wasteful and could be eliminated, with resulting cost savings. The upstream implications of reaching consensus are extraordinary.

Because the budget crisis is really a crisis, it behooves physicians to answer the waste question as rapidly as possible. Without an answer, there is no hope that an appropriate policy process for reining in health care costs will be identified. Physicians need to speak with one voice. Is there sufficient clinical waste to help address the federal budget deficit? If the answer is yes, physicians must be prepared to act quickly. If the answer is no, physicians must ensure that society understands the value of increasing health care expenditures more quickly than GDP growth, so that society can decide how much, if any, rationing will be necessary.

## References

1. Aaron HJ, Schwartz WB. *The Painful Prescription: Rationing Hospital Care.* Washington, DC: The Brookings Institution; 1984.

2. Cutler DM. *Your Money or Your Life: Strong Medicine for America's Healthcare System.* New York, NY: Oxford University Press; 2004.

3. US Congressman Paul Ryan. Issues: health care. http://www.roadmap.republicans.budget.house.gov/Issues/Issue/?IssueID=8516. Accessed July 11, 2011.

4. The New York Times. Arizona cuts financing for transplant patients. http://www.nytimes.com/2010/12/03/us/03transplant.html?_r=1&adxnnl=1&hpw=&adxnnlx=1308060528-LxRlgUvK+q8/7ImNDyMy1g. Accessed June 14, 2011.

# Can the Patient-Centered Outcomes Research Institute Become Relevant to Controlling Medical Costs and Improving Value?

*Robert H. Brook, MD, ScD*
JAMA, *November 9, 2011—Vol. 306, No. 18, pp. 2020–2021*

One result of health care reform legislation was establishment of the Patient-Centered Outcomes Research Institute (PCORI).[1] This relatively generously funded institute is intended to provide support for research that "helps people make informed healthcare decisions and allows their voice to be heard in assessing the value of healthcare options."[2] This kind of research "assesses the benefits and harms of preventive, diagnostic, therapeutic, or healthcare delivery system interventions to inform decision-making, highlighting comparisons and outcomes that matter to people."[2]

Research that the PCORI funds will not find the vaccine to cure cancer, the medication to eliminate obesity, or the treatment to cure Alzheimer disease. But the PCORI's research is important. This research can help physicians and patients decide which of multiple tests or therapies is slightly better or no different in terms of its effects on patients with specific symptoms or diseases. PCORI research can help to determine how the delivery of health care can be improved, perhaps by altering the way that teams of health professionals are assembled, or the ways that e-mail or telephone communication are used to deliver care.

Collecting detailed data about the cost of interventions being compared is not within the PCORI's scope, even though value, which most individuals believe includes cost, is central to the institute's mission. An example from past research brings the effect of this decision into sharper focus. More than 40 years ago, the US government funded the RAND Health Insurance Experiment (HIE).[3] Its purpose was to test whether patient cost sharing affected health care use, quality, health status, and cost of care. The HIE was so large that both the Secretary of Health, Education, and Welfare and the president had to authorize its funding. Indeed, the HIE was a page in the president's budget book. To replicate the HIE today might cost $1 billion—an amount similar to the PCORI's budget. Among the findings of the HIE that have been adopted is the use of patient cost sharing to incentivize patient and physician behavior.

What if the president, instead of signing off on the experiment, had said that the US government would pay for understanding how cost sharing affects health (which is what patients value) but that no cost data could be reported, and that the HIE's results could not be used to affect policy directly?

Within a few years, hundreds of studies funded by the PCORI will begin to appear in medical journals. Whether the studies focus on a test, a therapy, or a health delivery intervention, the results will be 1 of 2 types: (1) the test, therapy, or interventions being assessed led to small but statistically significant changes in health or another health outcome (some effects are likely to be small for an individual, but important when generalized to a large population)[4]; or (2) the alternatives being compared were deemed to be equivalent (all interventions produce different outcomes but small differences are difficult to detect, and powerful designs and large sample sizes are needed to detect them). However, regardless of the results of these studies, cost information almost certainly will not be included.

How might such studies be used by a patient and physician? Fast-forward to a potential conversation. Assume that the results are equivalent and the patient says to the physician: "I heard the distinguished leader of the Medicare program speak about the need for affordable health care. I want to do my part to keep Medicare costs down so give me the less expensive intervention, as long as my health is not impaired as a result." Other than scratching his or her head, how can the physician determine which of the 2 therapies would turn out to be less expensive either for the patient or for the system? If the results of the interventions showed a difference and the patient, who has a high deductible health plan, wants to know whether it is worth paying for X vs Y, how will the physician respond?

To the patient and the health system, value should mean both health and cost. For example, some employed individuals with chronic disease decreased their use of statins and antihypertensive medications in response to small increases in co-payment. This outcome would not have occurred if the patient's share of the cost of the medication were not important.[5] But in the absence of data about the cost of the intervention, it is impossible to inform patients about the effects of the trade-off they are making. So what can be done?

A scientific and political case could be made to amend health care legislation to require that cost be included in the studies that the PCORI funds. But in the current political environment, such a move could place the institute at grave risk of being defunded.

The research community could reject the policy of excluding cost by not applying for and not accepting funding under the conditions established by the PCORI. There is precedent for this kind of stance. For example, the federal government funds some important work by contract with the proviso in some contracts that the work cannot be published.[6] This condition could be considered analogous to excluding cost data in the PCORI studies. To their credit, many researchers and institutions do not apply for, or accept, federal monies under such conditions.

Medical journals choosing to publish the PCORI-funded research that does not include cost data could encourage authors to consider including comments about the potential implications of cost in clinical decision making in the discussion section of the article. The journals could also ensure that an accompanying editorial discusses cost implications.

Another approach might be to establish an institute for value-based health care, governed with complete independence from its sponsors. Private industries and foundations both have interests that might motivate them to fund such an institute. After an article based on the PCORI-funded research was published, investigators and analysts at the institute for value-based health care would conduct a cost analysis, which could be made available in the public domain.

With these approaches, the health care legislation governing the PCORI need not change, and the risk of defunding the PCORI would be averted. The resources for an institute for value-based health care could go farther because it need not fund the effectiveness part of many studies that would be relevant to health care professionals because those assessments will already have been funded by the PCORI. If such an approach proves feasible, perhaps this broader principle could be adopted: regardless of who funds the clinical research or where in the world it is conducted, it would be complemented by a cost analysis. This approach could apply to clinical trials funded by the National Institutes of Health, work performed by the US Preventive Services Task Force, or national coverage decisions made for the Medicare program—all of which ordinarily exclude cost considerations.

Many details would need to be resolved, but the world is truly flat when it comes to research. With cutbacks in health care being contemplated throughout the Western world, physicians and patients should be able to have fact-based conversations about value.[7] But to make that possible, creative ways must be found to address the limitations placed on work funded by the PCORI. Incorporating the cost and value perspective is essential so that the work of the PCORI can be clinically relevant and optimally used by patients and physicians.

# References

1. Patient Protection and Affordable Care Act, Pub L No. 111-148, 124 Stat 727,§6301.

2. Patient-Centered Outcomes Research Institute. Working definition of patient-centered outcomes research. http://www.pcori.org/assets/Summary-of-PCOR-Definition-Input-Opportunity-.pdf. Accessed September 7, 2011.

3. Newhouse JP; Insurance Experiment Group. *Free for All? Lessons from the RAND Health Insurance Experiment.* Cambridge, MA: Harvard University Press; 1993.

4. Roberts I, Shakur H, Afolabi A, et al; CRASH-2 collaborators. The importance of early treatment with tranexamic acid in bleeding trauma patients: an exploratory analysis of the CRASH-2 randomised controlled trial. *Lancet.* 2011;377(9771):1096-1101.

5. Goldman DP, Joyce GF, Zheng Y. Prescription drug cost sharing: associations with medication and medical utilization and spending and health. *JAMA.* 2007;298(1):61-69.

6. Brook RH. Health policy and public trust. *JAMA.* 2008;300(2):211-213.

7. Brook RH. The role of physicians in controlling medical care costs and reducing waste. *JAMA.* 2011;306(6):650-651.

# Two Years and Counting: How Will the Effects of the Affordable Care Act Be Monitored?

*Robert H. Brook, MD, ScD*
*JAMA, January 4, 2012—Vol. 307, No. 1, pp. 41–42*

In less than 2 years, all US citizens and legal US residents will have health insurance—except individuals who are willing to pay a penalty for not buying insurance. The United States is on the verge of joining the civilized world.[1] Of course, this outcome will occur only if, among other things, the US Supreme Court does not rule that the Patient Protection and Affordable Care Act is unconstitutional, if US and state governments can enact the necessary policies and regulations, and if the health insurance exchanges required to implement the law will work. Whether a proponent or a critic of this law, most will agree with the undeniable fact that a new era in US medicine and US health care begins in less than 2 years.

The key question is what potential measures should be monitored to determine both anticipated and unanticipated effects of the new law on the health of the US population.

The first measure of the law's success should be how much preventable mortality that is due to the health care system will be eliminated. Preventable mortality has many causes, ranging from personal behaviors to social determinants of health,[2] to poor inpatient and outpatient care.[3] Ways to assess preventable mortality have been available for many years.[4] It is time to develop a national sampling frame of deaths and to determine, almost on a real-time basis, the proportion of an individual's death that might have been prevented by better hospital care, better ambulatory care, or better personal behaviors. For example, a death from lung cancer in a patient who smoked could be attributed to smoking behavior, a stroke that occurred in a patient with inadequately controlled hypertension could be ascribed to poor ambulatory care, and an in hospital death from a central line infection could be attributed to poor hospital care. The goal of health care reform should be to drive the number and proportion of preventable deaths that are under the control of the medical care system (ie, deaths due to poor ambulatory or hospital care) as close to zero as possible. National baseline data regarding the numbers of preventable deaths are necessary to monitor the change in the preventable death rate over time.

The second measure of the law's success should be how many preventable hospitalizations are avoided. The United States has a large number of avoidable hospitalizations from ambulatory-sensitive conditions.[5] The rate of avoidable hospitalization varies across the nation by geographic area (poor neighborhoods have higher rates).[6] Examining the reason that a patient was admitted to the hospital—eg, uncontrolled diabetes or asthma—can help to determine whether the hospital admission could have been avoided with better outpatient care. Thus, the second goal of health care reform should be to drive the avoidable hospitalization rate from ambulatory-sensitive conditions to zero.

The third measure of the success of health care reform should be whether it increases to 100% the number of US residents who have access to a system of care. Loosely defined, this means that whether a patient needs emergency care, outpatient care, primary care, tertiary care, or an organ transplant, a coordinated system of care exists to ensure that the patient received the appropriate level of service and was able to access higher levels of medical care if needed. An organization that provides only emergency care without any arrangements for specific follow-up care does not represent a system of care. A health center that provides high-quality outpatient primary care but cannot arrange for subspecialty care or hospital care when needed is not a system of care. If a gynecologist needs to treat a woman with severe depression because she has no access to a mental health professional, she has no system of care. If the physician providing emergency care is not capable of reducing a complicated fracture but must attempt the reduction because no orthopedic surgeon is available, the patient with the fracture does not have a system of care.

This loose definition of a system of care does not require that a patient have a primary care gatekeeper or restricted access to a specialist. Rather, it requires that patients have a reasonable chance of receiving the level of care they need in a reasonably timely manner. Systems of care range from an accountable care organization to a health maintenance organization to the Veterans Affairs, but systems must be sufficiently organized, so patients with serious problems are not left to fend for themselves.

The fourth measure that can be used to monitor the health care reform act should be the cost of care divided by the number of individuals who are in a system of care. If health care reform is successful, the growth rate of health care costs for all US residents enrolled in a health care system should be reduced to the growth rate of the gross domestic product or less.

Other important variables could be assessed to monitor health reform, including years of life lost, disability-free years of life, functional health status, whether care is patient centered, or the appropriateness of surgery. However, concentrating on the 4 measures described in this article could help the nation to evaluate the facts and merits of this new health care system.

Implementation of health care reform may also have adverse or unpredictable consequences that should also be assessed and publicly reported. There are some concerns that health care organizations, nurses, and physicians will experience increased stress as more people access the health care system.[7] Accordingly, part of monitoring the success of health reform should be to measure the quality of how the workforce is treated. If health workers are increasingly pressured to become more efficient and productive, and this occurs in a manner that increases workplace injuries and stress, then health reform will not succeed. If the goal is to eliminate preventable mortality in patients, the number of workplace injuries in the health workforce needs to be reduced to zero.

In addition, if the law is successfully implemented, then individuals without insurance will include undocumented immigrants, some of whom have been living in the United States for many years, as well as individuals who have elected not to enroll in health care but instead pay a penalty. When an uninsured patient presents to an emergency department or physician's office, the physician will know that the patient is either an undocumented individual or somebody who has chosen to pay the penalty rather than pay for health insurance. How will that patient be treated? Until now, many patients without insurance seeking care were employed US citizens who were unable to acquire health insurance for medical or financial reasons. The law changes this dynamic. The issue will become whether individuals without insurance will be turned aside by health systems, including safety net systems such as county-run systems, or perhaps will be asked for payment before care is delivered. This possible effect should be carefully monitored, and the health consequences of such actions should be documented.

Moreover, in the United States, most of the large variation in life expectancy by race, ethnicity, social class, or neighborhood is not under the control of the medical system but rather is a consequence of the social determinants of health, such as acquiring a good education or obtaining a job with a livable wage.[6] All US citizens and legal residents should celebrate that lack of insurance will no longer be a barrier to obtaining needed medical care. However, because the health reform act absorbs energy, attention, and resources, the mortality gradients in US society by race, ethnicity, and social class may increase unless there are sustained investments in improving or eliminating those social determinants (eg, adequate support for public education).

Physicians should commit to participating in thoughtful and transparent evaluations of the new health law. As a beginning, baseline data should be collected and made available so that in the future, when other necessary changes to the law occur (health care legislation is never done), the evidence base for making those changes will be much stronger. Meanwhile, all Americans should celebrate that lack of health insurance in the United States will no longer be one of the causes of poor health.

## References

1. Patient Protection and Affordable Care Act, HR 3590, 111th Cong (2009).

2. Marmot M. Closing the health gap in a generation: the work of the Commission on Social Determinants of Health and its recommendations. *Glob Health Promot.* 2009(suppl 1):23-27.

3. Nolte E, McKee CM. Measuring the health of nations: updating an earlier analysis [published correction in *Health Aff (Millwood)*. 2008;27(2):593]. *Health Aff (Millwood).* 2008;27(1):58-71.

4. Dubois RW, Brook RH. Preventable deaths: who, how often, and why? *Ann Intern Med.* 1988;109(7):582-589.

5. Organisation for Economic Co-operation and Development. *Health at a Glance: 2011 OECD Indicators.* Paris, France: OECD Publishing; 2011.

6. Davison JD, Jones LS, Brown AF, Zingmond DS, Fink A, Washington DL. Community-academic partnering to monitor preventable hospitalizations and build community capacity for health advocacy and planning. In: 136th Annual Meeting of the American Public Health Association; October 25-29, 2008; Abstract 172929. http://apha.confex.com/apha/136am/webprogram/Paper172929.html. Accessed December 11, 2011.

7. West CP, Shanafelt TD, Kolars JC. Quality of life, burnout, educational debt, and medical knowledge among internal medicine residents. *JAMA.* 2011;9(306):952-960.

# Do Physicians Need a "Shopping Cart" for Health Care Services?

*Robert H. Brook, MD, ScD*
JAMA, *February 22/29, 2012—Vol. 307, No. 8, pp. 791–792*

Electronic medical records are being implemented throughout the US health care system. Incentives for implementation are being partially paid for by the US taxpayer. To receive implementation incentives, clinicians must demonstrate meaningful use—that is, the electronic medical record must be used to improve quality and must satisfy certain indicators.[1] What is missing from the definition of meaningful use is any direct measure of either value or cost. It is likely that introducing electronic medical records will improve quality on such dimensions as whether a vaccine is administered, measurement of blood pressure is taken, diabetes is better controlled, and admissions for poorly controlled diabetes are reduced.[2] However, in most systems there are no measures built into electronic medical records to help physicians control cost or even to know the cost of the care that they are providing.

Other organizations use computers to improve the purchasing experience, cost, and value of consumer products. Anyone who has shopped online has been presented with multiple ways to judge the quality of the product being purchased. There are ways to compare a given product with other similar products along specific dimensions, and to see what individuals who purchased the product thought about it. The assumption is that this information can help a consumer decide whether the product is worth the cost. However, the consumer's experience does not end with the description of the product's quality or efforts to encourage purchase of a better-quality product. Invariably the site has an electronic "shopping cart" that not only lists all the products that the consumer has put in the cart but also shows the cost of each one, as well as the total cost of everything in the shopping cart. The cart's total automatically updates whenever the cart's content is changed. In essence, on Internet sites, meaningful use means giving information to the consumer about the quality and the cost of a product in real time.

In the United States, the primary purchaser of medical care is the individual clinician, whether that is a physician or a nurse practitioner. Practitioners can access many sources to determine the quality of a test or procedure, but real-time cost data are not available anywhere. In this context, cost means what a typical patient who is insured by a typical company or by the government would be expected to pay for a given service. Cost includes both what the company or government paid and what the patient paid out of pocket. For example, if the insurance company paid the pharmacy $80 and the patient paid $8, the cost of this service is $88.

What if every time a practitioner used an electronic medical record system to order a procedure or test for a patient, an electronic shopping cart appeared, indicating how much that "purchase" would cost? What if at the end of the day the practitioner received a statement indicating precisely how much money he or she had ordered to be spent on behalf of patients? What would happen? Would anybody care? Some evidence suggests that providing this type of information to physicians may be helpful. For instance, in a study at one hospital, following the initiation of a weekly announcement informing the surgical house staff and attending physicians of the actual dollar amount charged to non–intensive care patients for laboratory services (ie, daily phlebotomy) ordered during the previous week, there were reductions in daily per-patient charges for laboratory services, with estimated cost savings of more than $50,000 over the course of the 11-week intervention.[3]

Perhaps the designers of computerized medical record systems should be advised that the records will be considered incomplete unless they contain information about the cost of the procedures, tests, or services that physicians are purchasing using the systems. How rapidly could the systems currently in use be modified to include such information? Perhaps it is time to begin making physicians and patients aware of what is being spent on a real-time basis, in a form with which they are comfortable.

Retail clinics,[4] which provide care for a limited number of acute and preventive conditions, post prices for their services. Patients can see what it will cost them to get a flu vaccination or to be evaluated for a urinary tract infection. But clinicians must do better than retail clinics, or at least as well. It should be possible to keep a running total of the costs for everything that a physician orders. For instance, every time a physician admits a patient to the hospital and orders the nurses to obtain vital signs every hour, or to collect intake and output, or to get the patient out of bed and walk the patient for an hour, a cost could be put into the record and into the shopping cart. Any time a physician ordered a laboratory test or procedure, the total in the shopping cart would be updated.

Once awareness about the cost of care on a real-time basis becomes part of the culture of medicine, perhaps the information could be used to increase the value of care and to control costs. At the very least, the presence of such information would be a wake-up call to physicians and nurse practitioners, helping them to understand just how much money is being spent on behalf of patients. The content and total cost of the shopping carts could be shared with patients so that they saw not only the list of tests and procedures and their results, but also the costs of those services in real time.

Once the cost data are collected from these shopping carts, there are many ways to present and analyze them. For example, it might be useful to compare physicians on the same clinic schedule, inpatient rotation, or in similar office practice settings. Such a comparison need not adjust for every difference in patient mix. Rather the purpose would be to develop a general picture of cost trends and spending patterns. Presenting the information in this way could produce a learning environment in which data could be used efficiently and effectively, potentially changing the production of value-based medicine.

On commercial websites, consumers are given incentives to purchase other products. For example, "Customers who bought this product also bought . . . " Or "Free shipping for purchases over $50." Such an approach might be adapted for the medical shopping cart. Analytical tools could be developed that assess the content of the shopping cart and suggest a different mix of services that would save X numbers of dollars or advise the physician "consumer" that 30 minutes of nursing time could be saved on an inpatient ward if care orders were modified in the following way. Such tools might indicate that efforts to reduce the total cost of a laboratory package should focus on a subset of 10 tests because they make up 90% of the cost as opposed to the other 80 tests that only make up 10% of the cost.

Consumers making Internet purchases are given multiple opportunities to consider whether they want to purchase a given product for a specified amount. The orders that physicians write cause patients and insurance companies to spend money, but physicians have no information about how much they have spent, how they might change the amount of money spent, or how they might provide a more cost-effective mix of services. The current system effectively shields physicians from cost information and hence prevents them from asking these kinds of questions. Maybe physicians should need to click twice instead of just once before placing an order just to increase the likelihood that the patient needs that service or test. Can health care learn from commercial Internet sites and translate the lessons into meaningful use criteria for medical records?

Any airline's site allows potential customers to search not just by schedule but by cost and schedule, and to narrow the schedule choices based on what the customer is willing or able to pay for a ticket. Changing the context to health care, does making a diagnosis in 3 weeks cost 3 times as much money as making the diagnosis in 4 weeks? If physicians and patients knew that it did, would they choose to change the time schedule for making the diagnosis in order to reduce costs?

Providing physicians with cost data in real time automatically as a part of the electronic medical record could make them better purchasers for their patients and provide better value. Given that patients in the future are likely to spend even more money out of their own pockets for premiums and the care they receive, increased attention to value may also increase patient satisfaction and enhance the likelihood that they will purchase only care that will improve their health.

# References

1. Centers for Medicare & Medicaid Services. CMS HER Meaningful use overview. https://www.cms.gov/EHRIncentivePrograms/30_Meaningful_Use.asp. Accessed January 12, 2011.

2. Hillestad R, Bigelow J, Bower A, et al. Can electronic medical record systems transform health care? Potential health benefits, savings, and costs. *Health Aff (Millwood)*. 2005;24(5):1103-1117.

3. Stuebing EA, Miner TJ. Surgical vampires and rising health care expenditure: reducing the cost of daily phlebotomy. *Arch Surg.* 2011;146(5):524-527.

4. Mehrotra A, Wang MC, Lave JR, Adams JL, McGlynn EA. Retail clinics, primary care physicians, and emergency departments: a comparison of patients' visits. *Health Aff (Millwood)*. 2008;27(5):1272-1282.

# Vision and Persistence: Changing the Education of Physicians Is Possible

*Robert H. Brook, MD, ScD*
J Gen Intern Med, *May 5, 2012—Vol. 27, No. 8, pp. 890–891*

More than 40 years ago, Margaret (Maggie) Mahoney,\* who was at that time a staff member at the Carnegie Corporation, had a series of meetings with distinguished professors of medicine, including John Beck of McGill, Julie Krevans of Johns Hopkins, James Wyngaarden of Duke, Austin Weinberger of Case, Hal Holman of Stanford, and Oliver Cope of Harvard. The purpose of these meetings was to address fundamental issues regarding the training of the future physician leaders of the United States. In the early 1960s, the emphasis on basic science training for physicians was entering a period of heightened intensity. The future of medicine was seen as tied directly to success in the wet laboratory. However, at the same time these stalwarts of American medicine and a young program officer at the Carnegie Corporation were discussing the need to produce a different kind of physician leader. These leaders would be trained in an emerging set of skills, including health policy analysis and health services research. These leaders entertained concepts that clearly were not part of wet bench medicine—for example, perhaps the purpose of treating patients should be to improve their functional status or health status, and thus physicians needed to be leaders in measuring health status and function. Perhaps measuring and improving quality of care was important. Perhaps one should explore and develop a host of new statistical and epidemiologic techniques to assess how they might be used in clinical medicine.[1,2,3]

The truly revolutionary aspect of these meetings was the desire to integrate population health and personal health. Before the meetings occurred, a physician interested in improving the health of a population or understanding something about how culture affected patient care and how that, in turn, affected health would normally depart for a school of public health after completing clinical training.[4] At places like Hopkins, the street that separated the School of Public Health from the School of Medicine was as broad as the DMZ separating North and South Korea. Everything one learned in clinical medicine, as well as the symbolic white coat and the stethoscope, was simply not acceptable in the School of Public Health. These leaders had a different vision. They

---

\*    Maggie Mahoney died on December 22, 2011.

believed that physicians could work in both clinical medicine and population health. To make this vision a reality meant defining a new field. Margaret Mahoney convinced the Carnegie Corporation and the Commonwealth Foundation to fund what would become the Clinical Scholars Program, thereby changing the face of medicine forever. She subsequently moved with the program to the Robert Wood Johnson Foundation, where she was the visionary who persuaded the foundation and each of its presidents to sustain funding of the Robert Wood Johnson Clinical Scholars Program. It may be the longest ongoing training program ever funded by a foundation.

The Foundation's support has continued without interruptions to this day, and the more than 1200 physicians who have gone through the Clinical Scholars Program have become the leaders of American medicine. They have held positions in government ranging from Surgeon General to Assistant Secretary. Some head state health departments or lead organizations such as the Joint Commission on Accreditation of Healthcare Organizations. Many are in academic departments including deans of both schools of medicine and schools of public health. The scope of their presence and influence cannot be overestimated. Indeed, it is hard to imagine modern American medicine without the leaders produced by the Clinical Scholars Program.

Due to the efforts of this new kind of physician, fields were redefined and new fields, such as measuring health status and quality of care and understanding how healthcare policies affect patient outcomes, were opened up. But the vision also included having these physicians remain active clinicians, and graduates of these programs, who assumed jobs ranging from foundation presidents to assistant secretaries in HHS, still manage to provide patient care in free clinics or make hospital rounds. In essence, Maggie Mahoney and the leaders with whom she met and who shared her vision, changed the culture of medicine. The walls between schools of public health and medical schools were torn down. Population health and the delivery of clinical services were no longer incompatible. Methodologies used in the social science became methodologies used in the clinical sciences. These new physician leaders who became accepted in both camps actually helped to merge the camps into one vision of health and health care for all.

But changing physician education requires more than a vision. For many of the past 40 years, Annie Lee Shuster, a program officer at The Robert Wood Johnson Foundation, used every skill in her armamentarium to convince the RWJ Foundation—its staff, its board, and its presidents as well as leaders of the Veterans Administration—to maintain the vitality of the Clinical Scholars Program. As a consequence, over those decades an extraordinarily diverse group of people has continued to allocate both financial and intellectual support for the Program. The results of this happy marriage of vision and persistence are many of the physician leaders of American medicine today.

Is there now an equally important change in physician education that needs to occur? The Internet and smartphones have changed the way we purchase consumer goods; crowd sourcing has changed the way ideas are vetted; and people organize to improve our products and services and even bring down governments. Social media has changed the way we find mates, choose hotels, and decide whether to try that new, pricy, restaurant. Communication has become 24/7. However, to a large degree, medicine both does not take advantage of and has not kept up with this instant feedback, always connected world. Medical education still focuses on what a physician does in face-to-face contact with the patient. Office visits and hospital rounds still dominate the culture of American medicine. Indeed, physicians still ask if it is acceptable for patients to contact their physician by e-mail, if a physician who is covering for another physician should provide the same quality of care for patients who are not hers as she does for her own, or whether physicians have any responsibility for following up on patients after they are out of sight—e.g., after they have been discharged from a hospital or been seen in the outpatient setting.

Perhaps it is time to ask a different set of questions. Should main-stream medical care be expanded beyond bankers' hours, following the basic pattern of retail stores and internet sites? Should patients play a more prominent role in managing their health? For example, instead of requiring patients to ask for their x-ray or lab results, perhaps they should be responsible for maintaining these records, producing them as needed for care. Should patients have more control of their health care? For example, why can't they get their blood pressure checked by using a machine in any drug store and then refill their prescription without contacting any doctor? Should patients be able to have blood drawn and have the results sent directly to them so that they can monitor their own illness? In short, how do we transform the vision of medicine from one in which physicians control the process, regulations dominate the playing field, and care is delivered at the convenience of health professionals to one in which patients are truly at the center?

Many small companies and physician entrepreneurs are tinkering with or investing seriously in producing a paradigm shift in the way care is delivered. In the new paradigm, the patient, not the physician, would be at the center of the universe. That shift would have enormous consequences, system-wide. For example, if the patient, not the doctor, were at the center of the universe, patients would not leave the hospital without an electronic copy of their records and all test results, written or printed in a manner they could understand and use to ensure that continuity of care became a reality. No patient who was discharged from the hospital and urgently needed physical therapy would need to wait days or weeks, watching themselves deteriorate, if they could arrange therapy immediately without waiting for somebody in authority to approve it.

The doctor of the future will need to partner with the patient in facilitating care and maintaining health. In this new world, a visit to a physician might be seen as a failure just as Internet providers believe that a visit to a store is a failure.[5] Perhaps in 20 years, seeing a physician will represent a failure rather than a revenue-generating event. Wouldn't it be nice if the education of physicians were guided not by how many hours need to be spent in the hospital or in outpatient care, but rather by what physicians need to do to reduce dramatically these activities by helping people improve and maintain health?

The need to prepare doctors for this paradigm shift is urgent. Forty years ago, nobody thought the Clinical Scholars Program would succeed; paradigms, as Maggie Mahoney demonstrated, can be changed.

## References

1. Brook RH. Health services research: is it good for you and me? *Acad Med.* 1989;64:124-130.

2. Brook RH, Kamberg CJ. General health status measures and outcome measurement: a commentary on measuring functional status. *J Chronic Dis.* 40 Supplement 1987;1:131S-136S.

3. Williams KN, Brook RH. Quality measurement and assurance: a literature review. *Health & Med Care Serv Rev.* 1978;1:1-15.

4. Brook RH. Having a foot in both camps: the impact of Kerr White's vision. *Health Serv Res.* 1997;32(1):32-36.

5. Brook RH. Disruption and innovation in health care. *JAMA.* 2009;302(13):1465-1466.

# Why Not Big Ideas and Big Interventions?

*Robert H. Brook, MD, ScD, FACP*
J Gen Intern Med, *December 2014—Vol. 29, No. 12, pp. 1586–1588*

Journals report evaluations of ideas or interventions intended to improve health care. For example, one article evaluated whether paying hospitals and physicians a bit extra for performance reduced mortality rates.[1] Another examined whether care coordination reduced hospitalization.[2] Others include a meta-analysis of whether the implementation of electronic medical records affects quality or cost,[3] an assessment of how free care in a chaotic medical system changes health status,[4] and an examination of whether a medical home that includes only technical management of a chronic disease improves the quality of care given to disadvantaged patients.[5]

These evaluations employ rigorous designs and sophisticated statistical methods; they take years to complete and publish. Very often, they yield negative results that can lead to dismissals of policies as ineffective. For example, pay-for-performance does not reduce mortality.[1] Discharge planning does not change readmission rates. Implementing electronic medical records neither saves money nor improves quality.[3] Changing the organization of practice to a medical home does not improve the quality of care for patients with diabetes.[5]

But let's consider for a moment. If we don't pay for performance, do we want to pay for non-performance? Does it make sense to provide no care coordination for people with chronic diseases? Does it make sense to provide chronic care in an uncoordinated fashion in which no one is in charge?

Any rational individual would answer no to these questions. So why is there a disconnect between basic common sense and the results of program evaluations? Perhaps it's because the policies being evaluated are too cautious to affect outcomes.

There are two basic approaches to developing health policies. The first, which is cautious and careful (a small idea and a small intervention or even a big idea and a small intervention), is more likely to be tested and implemented because institutions and professionals will not be threatened by the magnitude of the change. But this approach runs the risk of discrediting the concept that is being tested because what is being implemented is too limited, circumscribed, or piecemeal. For example, pay-for-performance (a big idea) that puts a small portion of provider compensation at risk (a small intervention), or electronic medical records (a big idea) that are implemented without a universal patient ID that can be accessed across platforms (a small intervention), will be less likely to improve either quality or reduce costs than those interventions that put 50% of compensation at risk or require a universal patient ID.

The second approach is disruptive and daring (big idea and big intervention). It can adequately test a concept, but the concept may be dismissed as infeasible (see Text Box.) What would society and physicians propose and accept if they were allowed to be creative and contravening regulations were set aside?

What if every patient with chronic disease who was discharged from the hospital had free access to their medications, the guidance of a health provider or community member who coached them daily to make sure they were doing the right things to stay out of the hospital, and access to a community online network of at least ten people who were paid to ensure that the patient never needed to be readmitted or never missed filling a prescription?

---

## What If?

1. All communities had a health plan that promoted an environment in which all people could thrive and a totally integrated set of social and health services to aid people in need.
2. Competency in understanding how health is produced was required of all graduates of junior and senior high school.
3. Educational and health policies were replaced with people policies that targeted the interaction between health and education as the way to improve a community's health. For example, improving educational outcomes by decreasing class size would be considered simultaneously with providing cognitive behavioral therapy to decrease stress produced by violence so that children will learn.
4. Most face-to-face physician visits were considered a failure of communication and technology, and such visits were replaced by video encounters, encounters with computers and people in the community, or self-directed care.
5. Global licensure of health professionals became a reality.
6. Medical expertise was shared so that by means of broadband/internet all people had immediate access, when needed, to world experts—without boarding a plane.
7. Obituaries contained information on whether the death could have been prevented by better medical care and/or whether the death was a good death (met expectations about growth, pain, and suffering).
8. Academic health centers put patients first and master clinician/teachers became the leaders of the institutions.
9. Expensive equipment was widely shared so that it could be used up before becoming medically obsolete.
10. Men and women understood the impact of an unplanned pregnancy on their lives, and if desired, received help in ensuring that all pregnancies are planned.

Why not test ideas and interventions that do them justice, such as those in the text box, that are actually worth evaluating because their potential effect could be substantial? For example, they will reduce cost growth not by 1%, but by 15%. They will extend quality-adjusted life not by days, but by a year. If the effect sizes were this large, one would not need sophisticated statistical analyses to prove that they were produced by the intervention. Simple evaluations would be all that was required.

If the intervention showed no obvious large effect, it could be discarded and the conceptual framework upon which it was based could be set aside. On the other hand, if powerful interventions showed the desired effects, then they could be made more efficient, and regulations could be revised to support these changes. That being said, it should be acknowledged that the success of even big interventions will likely depend on the circumstances or context in which they were implemented.

Currently, sophisticated analyses, understood by few, are being used to identify small positive effects. Those effects are probably also dependent on the context or site in which they were implemented and may not be reproducible.

Making marginal change wastes time, and the crisis facing the U.S. health system requires more than marginal change. We need to de-emphasize the current paradigm of examining interventions that we know will, at best, result in little change, and stop spending years trying to determine if the little impact is real. We need to stop wasting resources trying to implement minor interventions so that ten years later, a complicated statistical analysis will demonstrate a small effect that was significant at $p<0.05$.

Here is an alternative approach. The country should be divided into geographic areas defined by the density of the population and ranging from a few hundred thousand individuals to a few million. Each year we would devote 2 to 3% of U.S. health care expenditures in a few geographic areas to bold interventions designed to eliminate most of the major health problems identified in that area. The interventions would need to be supported by professionals and the community, and by both the public and private sectors.

The interventions would need to be culturally appropriate and ethically impeccable. If simple statistics demonstrated that a specific intervention met expectations, then a communication strategy employing mainstream and social media would be used to spread the news quickly to the world and to implement the intervention broadly. Of course, in doing this, one should not ignore the context in which the intervention was implemented and the context or circumstances to which the intervention was being spread. Even big ideas and big interventions need to be modified depending on context. For instance, large pay-for-performance incentives to increase the value of care given to people with chronic disease may not work in a community in which physician supply is so limited that physicians can only respond to emergencies.

Disruptive innovations are very risky—most fail—so they are less likely to be funded. But the Federal government and foundations need to focus on funding interventions that can produce substantial, meaningful results rather than on those that are faster to implement or less likely to fail.

Let's demand that we spend our intellectual capital and our limited resources on taking a real shot at eliminating the major problems that face us. For example, what would happen if a community and its health professionals formed an organization whose purpose was to maintain health and prevent premature death at an affordable cost? Would the community demand that equivocal and inappropriate care be eliminated? Would the community agree to end malpractice suits if evidence-based medicine were followed? Would the community agree to the goal of achieving 100% adherence to evidence-based medications and preventative services?

What would health professionals put on the table? Would they agree to allow a significant part of their compensation to be determined by the community? Would they agree to total transparency? Would they agree to involving the community as an equal partner in improving quality and eliminating waste, defined as services that are provided inefficiently or those that entail more potential health risk than health benefit?

Would this kind of conversation lead to a new system of delivering care and maintaining health that leapfrogs today's concept of affordable care organizations? Let's try to bequeath to our grandchildren a world in which we have identified and implemented a set of culturally sensitive, ethically appropriate interventions that harness the enormous advances in medicine achieved in the last century—that control costs and eliminate obesity, unplanned pregnancies, and avoidable readmissions for patients with chronic disease.

We face immense problems in health; solutions to them need to be commensurately big. Government and foundation money should be used to test and develop bold solutions. It should not be wasted on one more program that, at best, is expected to have a small impact.

# References

1. Jha AK, Joynt KE, Orav EJ, Epstein AM. The long-term effect of premier pay for performance on patient outcomes. *N Engl J Med*. 2012;366:1606-15.

2. Peikes D, Chen A, Schore J, Brown R. Effects of care coordination on hospitalization, quality of care, and health care expenditures among Medicare beneficiaries: 15 randomized trials. *JAMA*. 2009;3016:603-18.

3. Lubick Goldzweig C, Towfigh A, Maglione M, Shekelle PG. Costs and benefits of health information technology: new trends from the literature. *Health Aff*. 2009;28:2w282-93.

4. Brook RH, Ware JE, Rogers WH. Does free care improve adults' health?: results from a randomized controlled trial. *N Engl J Med*. 1983;309:1426-34.

5. Clarke RMA, Tseng CH, Brook RH, Brown AF. Tool used to assess how well community health centers function as medical homes may be flawed. *Health Aff*. 2012;31(3):1-9.

## About the Author

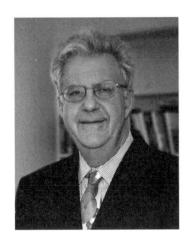

Robert H. Brook is a senior advisor and corporate fellow at the RAND Corporation, where he served for 19 years as vice president and director of RAND Health. He is also a professor of medicine and health services at the David Geffen UCLA School of Medicine and UCLA Fielding School of Public Health.

Brook led the Health and Quality Group of the $80 million RAND Health Insurance Experiment and was co-principal investigator of the RAND/UCLA Health Services Utilization Study, which developed appropriateness criteria for common medical procedures. He was also co-principal investigator on the only national study that has investigated, at a clinical level, how Medicare's prospective payment system affected the quality and outcome of acute hospital care.

Recognized as an international expert in the area of quality of care, Brook has published more than 560 scholarly articles. He is a member of the Institute of Medicine, the American Society for Clinical Investigation, and the American Association of Physicians. In 2005, Brook won the Institute of Medicine's Gustav O. Lienhard Award, cited as "the individual who, more than any other, developed the science of measuring the quality of medical care and focused U.S. policymakers' attention on quality-of-care issues and their implications for the nation's health." He has been awarded the Health Research & Education Trust (HRET) Trust Award, the David E. Rogers Award of the Association of American Medical Colleges, the Baxter Foundation Prize, the Rosenthal Foundation Award of the American College of Physicians, the Distinguished Health Services Researcher Award of the Association of Health Services Research, and the Robert J. Glaser Award of the Society of General Internal Medicine.